Accreditation in Primary Care

Towards Clinical Governance

EDITED BY

KIERAN WALSHE
NICOLA WALSH
THEO SCHOFIELD
CLARE BLAKEWAY-PHILLIPS

FOREWORD BY

LIAM DONALDSON
CHIEF MEDICAL OFFICER

RADCLIFFE MEDICAL PRESS

Radcliffe Medical Press Ltd
18 Marcham Road, Abingdon, Oxon OX14 1AA

British Library Cataloguing in Publication Data

A catalogue record for this book is available from the British Library.

ISBN 1 85775 322 4

Typeset by Multiplex Medway Ltd.
Printed and bound by TJ International Ltd, Padstow, Cornwall

Contents

Foreword

Quality is at the heart of the Government's modernisation strategy for the NHS. *The New NHS* and *A First Class Service* set out the components of a challenging programme for improving clinical quality in the NHS over the next five to ten years. Standards will be set by the National Institute for Clinical Excellence and National Service Frameworks, delivered locally through the development of clinical governance and monitored by the Commission for Health Improvement and the new NHS Performance Assessment Framework.

Clinical governance is the lynchpin of this quality improvement strategy, the vehicle for translating national standards and initiatives into meaningful improvements in patient care locally. It will be underpinned by lifelong learning and modern systems of professional self-regulation, and is reinforced by a new statutory duty of quality on NHS provider organisations.

Historically, although there has been good work on quality improvement in primary care (such as RCGP-led work to support the development of clinical audit), formal quality systems have in general been better developed in the hospital sector where there are clearer organisational structures to which they can be tied. But quality and clinical governance are just as important in primary care as they are in the acute sector. For the great majority of people, primary care is the face of the NHS with which they have the most regular contact – over 85% of all patient contacts happen here. And of course quality assurance of primary care and of commissioning will have a profound impact on the treatment patients receive when they are referred into secondary care.

NHS Executive guidance on clinical governance and on the development of PCGs emphasises the need for consistency in the broad approach to clinical governance across the NHS. There is though a need for implementation to be sensitive, recognising the importance of local ownership and the fact that different tools and techniques may be better suited to particular circumstances and different care sectors. Services need to explore the options and find out what suits them best.

Whatever methods are chosen, the imperitive for action is clear. Quality is at the heart of the primary care development agenda, just as much as for any other part of the NHS. The challenge is both to tackle cultural change, moving towards a more open and 'learning' system, and to help organisations and individuals find and use practical tools and mechanisms which can support work to make clinical governance a reality. Whether, in encouraging debate of specific quality improvements mechanisms or of the broader thinking behind them, this book is a valuable contribution to helping primary care organisations and those working within them approach the task of implementing clinical governance and improving quality at a practical level.

Professor Liam Donaldson
Chief Medical Officer
August 1999

List of contributors

Clare Blakeway-Phillips
Chief Executive
Aylesbury Vale Primary Care Group

Andrew Corbett-Nolan
Formerly Director of Development, Health Quality Service

Ann Foreman
Quality Manager
Northumberland Health Authority

John Hasler
Director
Edgecumbe Health Ltd

Sir Donald Irvine
President
General Medical Council

Peter Mitford
Director of Primary Care
Northumberland Health Authority

Theo Schofield
Senior Lecturer, Department of Public Health and Primary Care
University of Oxford

Nicola Walsh
Fellow, Health Services Management Centre
University of Birmingham

Kieran Walshe
Senior Research Fellow, Health Services Management Centre
University of Birmingham

Introduction:
the need for accreditation

Sir Donald Irvine

In the United Kingdom primary healthcare is based almost wholly on general practice. Since April 1999 all general practices have belonged to primary care groups. Questions of quality and accountability are high on their agenda as part of the new arrangements for clinical governance. This book on accreditation in primary care is therefore most timely.

For all of us, as patients, our family doctors and their practices are our normal link with the NHS and the usual way into specialist services. We want practices that are efficient, readily accessible, friendly and welcoming, and able and willing to provide us with a consistently good standard of professional care. We want our doctors to be technically competent and thoroughly up-to-date. We would like them to listen to us, to respect our views, to explain the management of illness as it unfolds in ways we can understand, and generally to be professional people who we can trust with our personal health affairs. When we need referral to hospital we rely on our family doctor to select skilled and able specialists in whom they, and therefore we, can have confidence.

In real life this is exactly what many patients experience, which is why good general practice is so well regarded. But for too many people expectation and reality are not the same. That part of general practice which provides indifferent or frankly poor care at its lower extreme is unacceptable by today's standards. Obviously in areas of deprivation and high workload it is more difficult to provide good care than elsewhere. Nevertheless it is a fact that, whatever the environment, good and poor care can and do exist alongside each other, in the same town, street and in the same practice. It persists today despite the many attempts by both the medical profession and successive governments to secure more consistent standards.

Now a new effort is being made to address the problem. The recent, highly publicised failures in medical care have brought a new sense of urgency in the medical profession to ensure that all patients get good care. At the same time, government has signalled its determination that the continuing tolerance of poor practice is not an option. So there is to be a new focus on quality. In each general practice the nurturing of a culture of continuous quality improvement, underpinned by competent quality assurance, is seen as fundamental, as the General Medical Council (GMC) has told every doctor in the booklet *Maintaining Good Medical Practice*.[1] Furthermore, there will have to be effective local arrangements for recognising and managing problems with the performance of individual clinicians when things seem to be going wrong. In general practice there is much practical experience to build on. Quality standards and internal and external peer review have been successfully and progressively developed and refined in teaching practices for a quarter of a century. So the question is not how to assess practice, but how to extend existing methods and knowhow to embrace the four-fifths of general practitioners who do not belong to a teaching practice.

Assuring good practice

Patients are critically dependent on the professionalism of their doctors, nurses and supporting staff, and on the collective responsibility assumed by practice teams for their standards and overall performance. Quality-assured practice is the key to giving patients the explicit assurances many now seek.

For doctors, the professionalism of the individual general practitioner is fundamental because so many clinical decisions are unsupervised. The GMC described the basic duties and responsibilities of all doctors in *Good Medical Practice*.[2] Essentially, each general practitioner must be competent, practise ethically, perform consistently well and protect patients from harm. The GMC has added recently that general practitioners must be able to demonstrate – on a regular basis – that they are keeping themselves up-to-date and that they remain fit to practise in their chosen field.

Complementing the doctor's personal commitment and responsibilities are the responsibilities of the practice team as a whole.[3] It is the team that is responsible for the environment for care – the practice building, equipment, staff and so on. Then there is care itself. Experience has shown that effective clinical teams are invariably well led, have a clear sense of direction and purpose, and are committed to their own blend of explicit values and standards. Such teams are open to new ideas, keen to learn and communicate well with patients and colleagues. They promote the professional development of each member. Effective clinical teams are inquisitive. They want to know how they are doing, whether they actually provide the standard of care they said they would. So they use the tools of quality monitoring – good records and data on performance, clinical and organisational audit, and regular personal appraisal. They are prepared to confront problems of individuals in the practice when they first arise, and see the resolution of these as a collective responsibility. Thus they help a colleague in difficulty before harm is done to patients, the colleagues or the practice, and they seek assistance when dysfunctional practice cannot be corrected by their own actions alone. It goes without saying that effective practices achieve this way of working by managing themselves well.

Practices that have this ethos are invariably keen to find out what others think about their care. They will use a range of strategies to discover what their patients think about their services, and will seek feedback from specialists and others to whom they refer patients. And, as experience with teaching practices has shown, they will want to know how they stand in relation to their peers.

Practice accreditation

This willingness to test against others is the starting point for the accreditation of practices as institutions, and the certification and revalidation of the professional credentials of individual practitioners.

The purpose is straightforward. Patients and carers – and employers and taxpayers – want to know for their own various reasons that general practices and their individual team members are practising a good and efficient standard of care, not just by their own lights but by recognised national standards. External review is therefore essential. External assessors, who should usually include members of the public as well as professional peers, will have several questions in mind. Do these practitioners know what they are trying to do, and what is expected of them? Do they sign up to and use explicit standards, and have they the means of finding out whether they apply them consistently, individually and collectively? Are they proactive, looking out for new opportunities and new ways of working? Do they learn from their experience, and so make and document changes that result in improvement?

The various forms of practice accreditation and personal revalidation described in this book reflect the means whereby such external reviews are currently carried out. Skilfully done, they are invaluable to a practice, as anyone who has experienced the process in a positive frame of mind will testify. They provide the kind of external stimulus and evaluation we all need. No doubt methods of internal and external review will develop quickly now, driven by the twin motors of local professional regulation and clinical governance.

At the end of the day, external review is only a means to an end. For patients, what matters is what happens when they visit their doctor, their practice and its team. Hence the central importance of maintaining the focus on the individual practitioner and the team – it is how they set about their professional business and how, day by day, they know they are giving good care that really matters. For patients, that is the ultimate determinant of quality.

1   General Medical Council (1997) *Maintaining Good Medical Practice*. GMC, London.
2   General Medical Council (1998) *Good Medical Practice*. GMC, London.
3   Irvine DH and Irvine S (1996) *The Practice of Quality*. Radcliffe Medical Press, Oxford.

Accreditation in primary care

Kieran Walshe and Nicola Walsh

Introduction

The past decade has been a time of enormous and sometimes overwhelming change for primary care in the UK. We have seen, for example, the introduction of a new contract for general practice in 1990, the development of GP fundholding and then a variety of other models of commissioning, such as total purchasing in the early 1990s, all as part of a general policy shift towards a 'primary care-led NHS'. More recently, we have seen moves by the current government to abolish fundholding, introduce primary care groups, and launch a raft of pilot initiatives in personal medical services (PMS), from salaried GPs to nurse-led primary care, under the new powers created by the Primary Care Act.[1] It is hardly surprising that there is a sense of perpetual revolution in primary care which, though often exciting for some, leaves others longing for stability and constancy of purpose.

One of the many changes we have seen in primary care in recent years is a growth in the importance attached to quality, and mechanisms for quality assurance and improvement. In particular, there has been a growing use of systems of accreditation, designed to measure practice in primary care against some form of external benchmark or standard, and use of the results to support changes and improvements in the quality of care for patients. Recent policy developments, particularly the introduction of primary care groups and the establishment of the concept of clinical governance,[2] have latterly done much to place the issue of quality centre stage in both primary and secondary care.

This book aims to provide a structured, critical review of the use of accreditation in primary care in the UK. First, it does so through chapters that describe the development of accreditation (Chapter 1) and outline an approach to evaluating accreditation programmes or understanding how they work and what they can achieve (Chapter 2). The book then provides four case studies (Chapters 3 – 6) of some of the most widely used approaches to accreditation in primary care in the UK, each structured to make it possible for readers to compare and contrast them for themselves. Finally, the last two chapters present the results of research evaluating one of these accreditation programmes (Chapter 7) and look forward to the future use of accreditation in primary care in the context of current policy developments, such as primary care groups and trusts and the introduction of clinical governance (Chapter 8).

To begin with, this chapter provides an introduction to accreditation, defining the concept and providing a succinct overview of its development, from origins in the USA at the start of this century to the present day.

Defining accreditation

Accreditation has been defined as 'a system of external peer review for determining compliance with a set of standard'.[3] In fact, the term 'accreditation' has been used to label a wide range of measurement or inspection processes in healthcare, and a number of other terms, such as certification, inspection, regulation and licensing, have also been used almost interchangeably. The semantics are not necessarily important, but the absence of clarity that this confusion of terms and ideas signifies does matter. We would suggest that accreditation systems are best recognised through the following five key characteristics:

- **review** of the performance or capacity to perform of a healthcare provider – usually an organisation such as a hospital or practice, but sometimes an individual practitioner;
- **external involvement** in the review, which is usually co-ordinated or led by some kind of statutory or professional agency and which often, although not always, involves peers – similar organisations or individuals to that undergoing accreditation, who have often themselves participated in the accreditation process;
- **standards** that define, to varying degrees of explicitness and measurability, the attributes of performance or capacity to perform that are to be assessed, and the values or circumstances that are to be expected;
- **measurement** of performance or capacity to perform against those standards, and the identification of areas where variances exist or where changes are needed;
- **report of results** of the process of review, which may contain an explicit judgement about the level of performance found and whether it reaches a certain accepted level, and may also offer a descriptive account containing conclusions and recommendations for action.

The definition cited at the outset of this chapter contained a curious omission: it said nothing about what accreditation is *for*. It might be thought at first that the purpose of accreditation would be self-evident, but it quickly becomes apparent that this is simply not the case. Only in the most general terms can it be said that a consensus about the purpose of accreditation exists, in that most systems are intended to maintain and improve standards of care. In fact, three main purposes for accreditation can be discerned:[4]

- **quality improvement** – using the accreditation process to bring about changes in practice that will improve the quality of care for patients;

- **informing decision making** – providing data on the quality of healthcare that various stakeholders, including healthcare funders, policymakers, managers, clinicians and the public, can use to guide their decisions;

- **accountability and regulation** – making healthcare organisations, which are usually professionally dominated, accountable to statutory or other agencies, such as professional bodies, government, patient groups and society at large, and regulating their behaviour to protect the interests of patients and other stakeholders.

But there are often important conflicts between these three goals, which an example may serve to illustrate. The standards and criteria against which performance or capability is assessed are central to any accreditation system. If the purpose of the process is quality improvement, then those standards and criteria should be challenging, able to identify opportunities for improvement in even the best practices, so that every accreditation visit results in a worthwhile set of recommendations that will bring about change and improvement. It may not matter whether the standards are particularly measurable, since their main value may be in identifying areas where opportunities for improvement lie, rather than in documenting current practice in detail.

However, if the purpose of accreditation is to inform decision making, then a quite different set of accreditation standards and criteria may be needed. Here, the key aim is differentiation – enabling those who will use the information to identify differences in performance among practices – so standards that most could meet, or that most could not meet, would not be very helpful. So the standards need to be capable of showing a broad range of performance from excellent practices (which might meet all or most of the standards) to poor practices (which might only meet a few of them). It is important that the differences in performance that the accreditation standards show are real and meaningful, rather than being a result of variations in the way that the assessors interpreted or applied them. So, in this case, the measurability of the standards (encompassing issues such as validity and reliability) is very important.

The third main purpose of accreditation – accountability and regulation – is likely to require different standards and criteria too. Here, the concern is likely to be focused on defining a minimum standard below which no practice should fall. The standards are therefore likely to be set at a level with which most practices can comply with ease, and only a few practices will have difficulty in demonstrating that they meet all the standards. Again, because the decisions taken on the basis of accreditation could be very serious, such as the implementation of sanctions or special measures to tackle 'failing' practices, the measurability of the standards is crucial to the accreditation process.

In other words, different purposes are likely to result in quite different sets of standards for accreditation. If an accreditation system is intended to serve conflicting purposes (or if the purpose is unstated and open to different interpretations), then the resulting standards will reflect that conflict and confusion.

The development of accreditation in healthcare

Accreditation has a long history in public services, and particularly in healthcare.[5] Box 1.1 provides a brief chronology. The first real healthcare accreditation system was developed in the USA just after the First World War, led by the American College of Surgeons, which was seriously concerned about standards of facilities and practice in acute hospitals, and much influenced by the ideas of scientific management that were popular at the time. The programme it established grew until, in 1951, a new organisation – the Joint Commission for the Accreditation of Hospitals – was set up to run it. Canadian hospitals also took part, and in 1959 a separate Canadian Council for Hospital Accreditation was established. In 1974, after some pilot work, a system of hospital accreditation was put in place in Australia, run by the Australian Council on Hospital Standards. For many years, these three anglophone countries were the only places where accreditation was used on a large scale, but more recently there has been an explosion of interest in accreditation internationally, with accreditation systems of various types being developed in France, Spain, the UK, Hungary, South Africa and many other countries. An international accreditation council is being established, and representatives of over 40 countries have been involved in its development.[6]

Box 1.1: The international development of accreditation in healthcare

1921   Hospital Standardisation Programme established by American College of Surgeons, following a highly critical national survey of hospital organisation and facilities.

1951   Joint Commission on the Accreditation of Hospitals established to take over running of US accreditation programme (later renamed Joint Commission on the Accreditation of Healthcare Organisations).

1959   Canadian Council on Hospital Accreditation set up to run national programme of accreditation in Canada (previously part of JCAH programme). Later retitled the Canadian Council on Health Facilities Accreditation.

1974   Australian Council on Hospital Standards founded, following long-standing interest in practice in Canada and the USA, to run accreditation programme in Australia (later renamed the Australian Council on Healthcare Standards).

1988/89   Development of Hospital Accreditation Programme and King's Fund Organisational Audit programme in the United Kingdom.

1990s   National accreditation programmes for healthcare organisations established or piloted in many other countries including France, Switzerland, Spain, Israel, Taiwan, Brazil, Hungary and South Africa.

We can only speculate at the reasons for the international interest in accreditation, and in other approaches to quality assurance and improvement in healthcare. It seems that societal changes (reduced trust in the professions, increased consumerism, rising expectations of healthcare, and so on) and healthcare system changes (increased technology, cost pressures, rising managerialism, and so on) have all played a part in creating an almost irresistible international movement towards greater oversight, regulation and explicit performance measurement in healthcare.

In the UK, a number of forms of accreditation in healthcare have existed for many years. For example, the Health Advisory Service, established in 1969, inspected services for the elderly, mental health and learning disabilities for almost three decades, and continues to exist in modified form today. The Mental Health Act Commission fulfils a statutory remit to oversee some aspects of mental health services. The United Kingdom Central Council for Nursing, through bodies in England, Wales, Scotland and Northern Ireland, assesses the suitability of healthcare organisations to provide or participate in nurse training. The medical Royal Colleges undertake inspections to accredit hospitals for the training of junior doctors. Health authorities undertake statutory inspections of nursing homes for the purposes of registration. But most of these long-standing accreditation and inspection programmes have been isolated initiatives, focused on particular care groups, services or professions, with rather narrowly defined aims and objectives.

It was not until the late 1980s that healthcare accreditation in the UK began to move beyond this rather piecemeal and fragmented approach, towards a more integrated model like that already used elsewhere. Two major hospital accreditation programmes were developed in the late 1980s and early 1990s. First, the King's Fund supported the creation of an organisational audit programme, drawing on the Australian experience of accreditation. Secondly, the South Western Regional Health Authority funded the establishment of a hospital accreditation programme, aimed mainly at smaller, community hospitals, which developed a national reputation in this area. Both programmes have been quite widely taken up and both continue to exist, albeit in modified form, today. Their development sparked a wider interest in the ideas of accreditation, with pathology laboratories, therapy professions, accident and emergency departments, other NHS regions, non-clinical services and others all starting to produce their own versions of accreditation.

For many years, the Department of Health took little interest in the use of accreditation, and seemed even to actively discourage its development, perhaps because of fears about the impact of a new inspectorate and the problems or embarrassments it might produce for civil servants and ministers. However, that policy gradually changed to one of mild encouragement during the 1990s. Reorganisation in the health service created much greater local autonomy, weakened traditional lines of management responsibility and review, and meant there was a need for new forms of control and accountability, which accreditation might meet. Experience in other settings (particularly education, where the Office for Standards in Education had been created) may have helped to dispel concerns about the political consequences of some form of accreditation. Even so, national policy did little to promote the development of accreditation until very recently.

The publication by the new government in 1997 of a White Paper *The New NHS: Modern, Dependable* marked a turning point in policy terms.[1] For the first time, proposals were presented for the development of a national inspectorate tasked with assuring the quality of healthcare in the NHS. To be called the Commission for Health Improvement, the new body will undertake periodic inspections of all NHS trusts, and will be responsible for reviewing local action to implement national guidelines on clinical practice.[2] The Commission will be, in effect, a national inspectorate for the NHS, and is likely to use some form of accreditation process as the basis for its inspections. Alongside other proposals in the White Paper, this represents a remarkable move towards greater central direction and control over standards and quality in the NHS, and towards a more corporate and managed form of clinical practice.

Even from this brief review, it is clear that accreditation is widely used, both in the UK and internationally, as an approach to managing and improving quality in healthcare. Moreover, interest and activity appears to be growing rather than receding, with new accreditation programmes being established in many countries. There is great variation in how accreditation is implemented, with differences in almost every area – who manages the programme, what sort of standards are used, who undertakes the process, how it is done, how the results are used, and so on. This heterogeneity should offer an opportunity to learn from the experience of different approaches but, in practice, evaluations of accreditation programmes have been rare, and comparative evaluations across systems or even across countries have been even rarer.[7] For this reason, our understanding of the costs and benefits of accreditation is very limited. The advocates of accreditation have little rigorous research evidence with which to demonstrate its effectiveness in achieving its objectives.

It is also evident that in most countries, secondary care services have been the primary focus of accreditation activity, with accreditation programmes in primary care developing rather later, if at all. In the USA, Australia and Canada, the accreditation bodies described earlier all began with titles that focused explicitly on hospital accreditation, and all changed their names to reflect a wider remit as they began to work outside the hospital setting. This focus on secondary care in accreditation may simply reflect the predominance of secondary care in most healthcare systems, but it may also have been influenced by a perception that secondary care services are more straightforward to accredit because of their better-defined organisational structure and arrangements, and by the belief that the effects of poor quality in secondary care may be more significant for patients because of the complexity and risk inherent in much acute care. Primary care has begun to be seen as more important, both as a provider of an increasing range of healthcare services in the primary care setting and as a gatekeeper to expensive secondary care services, and this has led to a growing interest in accreditation in primary care.[8]

Accreditation in primary care

The term 'primary care' is sometimes used to describe almost all health services provided outside the acute or hospital sector – including community health services, primary medical care, community mental health and learning disability services, rehabilitation and elderly care, and even community hospitals.[8] The shift of traditionally acute health services out of hospitals and into community settings blurs the boundaries still further. We have taken primary care to mean those health services that tend to be the first point of contact for patients seeking health services, provided in a community setting, by healthcare professionals who are generalists rather than specialists, in ways that promote continuity of care over time or longitudinal contact between patients and healthcare professionals.[9]

If this definition of primary care is used, accreditation has not been widely developed or used in primary care, even in those countries that have had established accreditation systems in secondary care for many years.[5,8]

It was noted above that accreditation has tended to develop first in the hospital setting, and for the establishment of accreditation in community and primary care services to then follow, but this has not been the case in the United Kingdom. In fact, it can be argued that the earliest national accreditation activity in the UK took place in primary care, led by the Royal College of General Practitioners, and that the rather more widely known UK secondary care accreditation programmes were only subsequently established.

In 1980, the Royal College of General Practitioners set up a working party to 'devise a method of assessing the performance of established general practitioners in the setting of their own practices', and a year later it published a report called *What Sort of Doctor?*, which set out, for the first time, a series of statements about the standards of practice and performance to be expected from a general practitioner. Under four main headings – clinical competence, accessibility, ability to communicate, and professional values – the report defined 36 standards, and offered a set of measurement criteria designed to support assessment against the standards.[10]

Between 1982 and 1985, a further working party refined the criteria, undertook field testing in three faculties of the College, and undertook an evaluation. It concluded that the tool that had been developed could be used in awarding membership or fellowship of the College, in appointing GPs and practices to train future practitioners, to develop similar standards for other primary care staff and functions (such as practice management) and to spread good practice between faculties and within the profession. These proposals were not greeted with universal enthusiasm, and may have seemed too radical for many in the profession. As a result, they were not generally adopted and much of the momentum of these pioneering efforts was lost.

Viewed in retrospect, *What Sort of Doctor?* can be seen to have been a truly far-sighted and creative initiative that has influenced quality improvement activities in general and accreditation especially, not just in primary care. A number of potential uses of the tool were envisaged by the working party in their report, and all of them have since come to pass. For example, fellowship of the College is now awarded through this kind of assessment tool, and work is in progress on a similar process to award membership, as they suggested. Training practice status is now given on the basis of practice visits and assessments using a set of criteria similar to those developed for *What Sort of Doctor?*, just as the working party proposed. Accreditation programmes have now developed that address the performance of other professional groups, such as nurses and practice managers, and of practices as a whole, which again the working party predicted. There are now several accreditation-based activities or initiatives in primary care in the UK, many of which owe something in design or development to the influence of *What Sort of Doctor?*, and a number of which have been set up by various faculties of the Royal College of General Practitioners. A summary of some of the main initiatives is given in Box 1.2.

Box 1.2: Accreditation programmes in primary care in the UK

King's Fund Organisational Audit (KFOA) programme in primary care

The King's Fund first established a pilot programme of hospital organisational audit in the late 1980s, drawing on the experience of accreditation in Australia but developing standards for the UK through a widespread consultation with interested groups and not linked to a formal accreditation award. It then moved to establish similar accreditation programmes for other healthcare organisations, including community hospitals and health authorities. It established a primary care accreditation programme in 1993, and has since undertaken organisational audits of over 250 practices. It has now been renamed the Health Quality Service.[11]

continued

Health Services Accreditation (HSA) programme in primary care

Health Services Accreditation is an NHS agency established by the South Thames Regional Health Authority in the early 1990s to take forward a regionally based programme of standards development. It began by working on standards in a number of clinical areas or specialities, and developed a portfolio of accreditation instruments. In 1997, HSA published draft standards for primary care in two areas – the organisation of primary care, and the management of a selected group of 17 common conditions – for consultation. No field use of the standards has been undertaken.[12]

Joint Committee on Postgraduate Training in General Practice (JCPTGP) – training practice assessment

The accreditation of practices to undertake the training of doctors who want to become general practitioners has been in operation since this form of vocational training was introduced in the mid-1970s. JCPTGP sets same national standards, which are then adapted by regional postgraduate training organisations that organise visits to practices who apply for training practice status. On some estimates, up to 25% of all practices have training practice status, so this accreditation system is by far the most widely used approach in the UK.[13]

Royal College of General Practitioners – team-based practice accreditation programme

The RCGP team-based accreditation programme was developed by a College working party from 1994 to 1996, and was piloted during 1997 with 12 practices in one health authority, though it has yet to be used more widely. It uses a set of standards and an assessment process that are managed locally, by the health authority, local medical committee, clinical audit group or other local organisation.[14]

continued

Royal College of General Practitioners – fellowship by assessment scheme

In the past, fellowship of the RCGP was awarded, on nomination by colleagues, largely for contributions to research, teaching or national developments. In 1989, the RCGP introduced a new route to fellowship, based on excellence in practice. Drawing on the experience of *What Sort of Doctor?*, a set of standards and an assessment process managed by faculties of the College were developed. So far, just over 100 members of the College have become fellows by this route.[15]

Royal College of General Practitioners – quality practice award

Developed by the north-east Scotland faculty of the RCGP, the quality practice award draws on the experience of *What Sort of Doctor?* and fellowship by assessment, but is focused on the whole practice team rather than just the doctor or doctors. It uses a set of standards and an assessment process which again is undertaken by the faculty. So far, only a few practices in north-east Scotland have received the award, but there are plans to offer it more widely.[16]

Conclusions

The context and nature of primary care presents different needs and challenges for accreditation programmes which often draw on the experience gained in secondary care settings.

First, accreditation is often (as the original title of the King's Fund's programme suggests) focused primarily on organisational issues, to do with the structures and systems in place to provide healthcare. This may work well in hospitals, where there are well-defined organisational structures and systems to measure. But in primary care, the organisational structures are often justifiably simpler, more fluid, less explicitly defined and less clearly bounded. It may be more difficult to set meaningful standards in these areas, and doing so may be less necessary.

Secondly, there is great diversity in primary care, some of which reflects important differences in the context for care and the population served, and some of that results from the many different configurations of practice that exist. This justifiable diversity may make setting meaningful standards difficult, since what is appropriate for an affluent, semi-rural population may not be so for a highly mobile, deprived population in an inner city. What might reasonably be expected of a large, multi-partner group practice in purpose-built premises may be an unreasonable or inappropriate demand on a single-handed practice in a converted house. Setting standards that act as a common benchmark for practice, but which do not force an unnecessary uniformity and reduce justifiable diversity, is far from easy.

Furthermore, hospitals are large organisations, and there are relatively few of them. General practices are much smaller, and there are many more of them. These differences of scale also present challenges for accreditation programmes. Large hospitals have a critical mass of expertise and resources that enables them to take on the task of preparing for accreditation and implementing recommendations that arise from assessment. Practices may be much more constrained in both their ability to prepare adequately for accreditation, and their capacity to manage the resulting change agenda. While an accreditation programme working with hospitals can generally build close, ongoing relationships with the organisations it is accrediting, and develop some knowledge of them over time, it is probably not possible to do this when working with a very large number of individual general practices in primary care.

1   Department of Health (1997) *The New NHS: Modern, Dependable.* The Stationery Office, London.

2   Department of Health (1998) *A First-Class Service: Quality in the New NHS.* Department of Health, London.

3   Scrivens E (1995) *Accreditation: Protecting the Professional or the Consumer?* Open University Press, Buckingham; p.9.

4   Klein R and Scrivens E (1993) The bottom line. *Health Service Journal.* **103** (5380): 24–6.

5   Sketris I (1988) *Health Service Accreditation – An International Overview.* King's Fund Centre, London.

6   International Society for Quality in Health Care (1997) *International Standards and Accreditation for Health Care: Feasibility Paper.* ISQua, Victoria, Australia.

7   Scrivens E (1997) Assessing the value of accreditation systems. *European Journal of Public Health* 7: 4-8.

8   Scrivens E and Blaylock P (1997) *Developments in Accreditation in Primary Care.* ISQua, Victoria, Australia.

9   Fry J and Horder J (1994) *Primary Care in an International Context.* Nuffield Provincial Hospitals Trust, London.

10 Royal College of General Practitioners (1985) *What Sort of Doctor? Assessing Quality of Care in General Practice.* Royal College of General Practitioners, London.

11 King's Fund Organisational Audit (1996) *Primary Health Care: Organisational Standards and Criteria.* King's Fund, 1996, London.

12 Health Services Accreditation (1997) *Standards for Primary Care Organisation: A Consultative Draft.* Health Services Accreditation, Battle, East Sussex.

13 Irvine D and Irvine S (1996) *The Practice of Quality.* Radcliffe Medical Press, Oxford.

14 Royal College of General Practitioners, Practice Accreditation Working Party (1997) *Pilot of Primary Health Care Team Based Accreditation: Progress Report.* Royal College of General Practitioners, London.

15 Royal College of General Practitioners, Vale of Trent Faculty (1997) *Fellowship by Assessment – Criteria (FBA8).* Royal College of General Practitioners, Nottingham.

16 Royal College of General Practitioners, North East Scotland Faculty (1997) *Quality Practice Award (Version 2).* Royal College of General Practitioners, Aberdeen.

2

Evaluating accreditation programmes in healthcare

Kieran Walshe and Nicola Walsh

Introduction

In view of the widespread adoption and development of accreditation in healthcare, described in Chapter 1, surprisingly little attention has been paid to evaluating accreditation initiatives and particularly to measuring their impact on the quality of care. In recent years, the rise of 'evidence-based healthcare' has done a great deal to sensitise clinicians, policy makers and others to the need for new healthcare interventions to be rigorously researched before they are introduced. The effectiveness of new and existing diagnostic and therapeutic interventions is increasingly challenged, and precedent and personal opinion are slowly giving way to scientific enquiry and research evidence as determinants of clinical practice.

Inevitably, the same set of questions to do with the effectiveness of interventions is starting to be applied to other forms of innovation in healthcare delivery, and not just to new clinical techniques or pharmaceuticals. Organisational interventions, such as accreditation, should be evaluated just as carefully and rigorously before they are introduced, and their adoption should be informed by the findings from such research. While the methods by which organisational interventions are evaluated may differ from the highly quantitative, experimental approach used to assess the effectiveness of clinical therapies, the challenge remains the same – does it work?

For accreditation programmes, the question 'does it work?' poses a string of other questions in turn. In order to assess the effectiveness of accreditation, we first have to develop a clear understanding of the objectives of the programme and the dynamics of the accreditation process. To this end, some form of framework for evaluation is needed, particularly if the intention is to compare and contrast different accreditation programmes which may be structured in quite different ways.

Developing a framework for evaluation

Box 2.1 sets out seven issues that are important considerations in developing or selecting an approach to accreditation, some of which are drawn from a useful taxonomy of such systems.[1] For each area or dimension listed in the box, a series of questions about the design and application of any approach to accreditation can be posed. Interpreting and using the answers that might be provided is not necessarily straightforward, and it would be unwise to label any particular configuration as 'better' than any other. Rather, we would suggest two criteria by which an assessment of the likely value of an accreditation system could be made, using data in these seven dimensions: internal consistency and contextual appropriateness.

Internal consistency

It would be legitimate to expect that for any particular accreditation system, the results of an assessment using this framework are internally consistent. In other words, the design of the standards and the methods of assessment should be consistent with the overall purpose of the accreditation programme, and so on. If obvious conflicts or difficulties are revealed, then their impact on the application of the accreditation programme should be considered.

Contextual appropriateness

Secondly, it is important that the appropriateness of the accreditation system to the context in which it might be used is discussed. This might involve a consideration of whether, in each of the areas identified in the box, the description of the accreditation programme fits the local setting. Again, discrepancies or likely difficulties should be highlighted.

Box 2.1: Issues to consider in developing or selecting an approach to accreditation

1. Purpose
2. Participation and coverage
3. Standards
4. Assessment methods
5. Presentation and dissemination of results
6. Impact and follow-up
7. Costs

Purpose

It was noted earlier that the purpose of accreditation programmes can vary, and that three main objectives – quality improvement, informing decision making, and providing accountability or regulation – could be identified, and that while these objectives could be complementary, they might also conflict. The purpose of any accreditation programme needs to be explicit, because without clearly stated objectives, it is difficult to make meaningful decisions about many other important issues (such as the design of standards, the methods of assessment, the use and dissemination of results, and so on). Evaluating an accreditation programme is difficult if we cannot identify objectives against which its performance can be measured. It may be helpful to consider the completeness and clarity with which the purpose of an accreditation programme is expressed, and to explore the consistency of and potential for conflict between its objectives.

Participation and coverage

Most accreditation programmes are voluntary, though some are mandatory. Voluntary accreditation programmes attract a self-selected population of participants, which is unlikely to be representative of all potential participants. It is self-evident that those organisations or individuals who take part are more likely to be those with an interest in quality improvement or a questioning, evaluative culture. Those who do not take part are more likely to be those for whom participation might be difficult or demanding, or those who are uninterested in quality improvement. In this way, it can be argued that voluntary accreditation programmes tend to focus on those organisations or individuals who are already likely to be providing high-quality healthcare, and may be less likely to involve those where quality problems are present.

On the other hand, mandatory accreditation programmes force participation on the reluctant and unwilling, and may mean that some participants are effectively involved under duress. In these circumstances, their commitment to the purposes of the accreditation programme, and willingness to co-operate and work with it, may be limited. The different advantages and disadvantages of voluntary and mandatory participation need to be seen in the context of the purposes of the accreditation programme.

In voluntary accreditation programmes, the incentives to take part and barriers to participation become very important. Incentives can include financial and competitive benefits, such as access to additional funding or the award of new contracts. The recognition by peers and patients that goes with accreditation may also be an incentive to take part. If the accreditation programme is a constructive force for change and improvement within the organisation, this too can be a useful incentive to participate. However, the incentives for organisations to take part in voluntary accreditation programmes can be quite weak, relying largely on individual enthusiasm and interest, goodwill towards the accreditation programme and its sponsoring organisation, and a sense of individual or organisational duty.

There are many potential barriers to participation, which may counter the incentives discussed above. Taking part may be resource intensive, requiring an investment of time, effort and funds that the organisation is not willing to commit. Accreditation may not fit well with other quality-improvement activities already under way, and may simply be a low priority when set against other, more urgent organisational demands.

Whether it is voluntary or mandatory, it should be possible to estimate the coverage of an accreditation programme – what proportion of potential participants have actually taken part. In mandatory programmes, participation will usually be at or near 100%, but voluntary programmes usually have much lower coverage. Very low coverage might be expected in pilot or experimental programmes, but in established accreditation systems such low take-up could be seen as an indication of limited support. Once again, the coverage of the accreditation programme needs to be seen in the context of its purpose.

Standards

Standards are at the heart of every accreditation system. They reflect the purpose of accreditation, embody the concept of performance it addresses, and form the foundation of the assessment method and results. There are four main dimensions on which the nature of the standards specified and used in an accreditation programme might be assessed: their level, content, derivation and measurability.

The level at which standards are set, or their stringency, is concerned with how difficult they may be for participants in the accreditation programme to meet. Minimal standards represent a lower limit to acceptable practice, and define care in ways that all, or almost all, organisations should be able to meet. Normative standards represent the patterns of practice that might be found in the average organisation, and are likely to be met by some and not by others. Optimal or ideal standards are set at a level that represents a challenge even for the best organisations, and which may be unattainable for some.

The content of the standards used in an accreditation programme refers to their scope, structure and specificity. It is clearly not feasible for any accreditation programme to be wholly comprehensive, setting standards for every possible area of practice or organisation, and all make choices both about how much to attempt to cover and what to include or exclude, which together can be termed the scope of the standards. The structure of the standards can also vary. For example, some accreditation programmes use organisational structures (such as departments or specialities) to subdivide standards, while others use particular healthcare processes (such as in-patient care, or day surgery) and others again are structured around particular dimensions of performance. Even when accreditation programmes address the same issues, they can vary in how specific they are about the nature of expected performance. For example, one might require that a policy or procedure exists, while another might specify some elements to be contained in that policy or procedure.

The derivation of standards in accreditation is a difficult and increasingly controversial matter. Traditionally, accreditation standards have been set through a process of consultation and consensus development, in which a range of interested parties have been brought together to agree standards, which have then been iteratively revised through wider consultation. There are a number of drawbacks to this approach, such as the risk that decisions can be led by particularly influential members of the group, and the potential that resulting standards can simply reinforce current practice rather than challenging it if need be. But, most obviously, this approach makes at best indirect use of research evidence (via the perspectives of group members), and the professional consensus standards that emerge can be at odds with the findings from research. However, in many areas in which accreditation standards are set, there is little research evidence on which to draw, which can be seen as either a justification for using consensus development methods or a reason for not setting standards in such areas at all. There are other issues to consider in connection with the derivation of accreditation standards, such as the rigour and explicitness of whatever methodology is used to develop them, and the likelihood that it will promote ownership of the standards among participants in the accreditation programme. Some accreditation programmes countenance little or no variation in the standards once they are developed – there is no provision, for example, for local organisations to add their own standards, or to alter existing standards. Others, often with a view to securing greater ownership, regard their standards as a common core on which to build, and encourage local variation.

A final but crucial concern is the measurability of the standards used in any accreditation programme. It might be assumed, given the nature of accreditation, that all standards would need to be measurable, but sometimes standards address important but intangible aspects of practice. If areas in which measurement is difficult are excluded, then the resulting standards could be seriously incomplete. On the other hand, if the results of assessment against standards are used in decision making, then there will clearly be a need for standards to be objectively measurable, with satisfactory validity and reliability.

Assessment methods

Accreditation usually involves some form of assessment, with external involvement, against the accreditation standards. However, the data sources and methods used for assessment, and the people responsible for making the assessment, may vary considerably. Most accreditation programmes draw on a range of data sources, including a written submission from the organisation to be accredited; special data collection exercises (such as specific audits), which they are required to undertake; and visits by a team of assessors, which can be used to gather data from staff, patients and other sources.

The degree of external involvement in the assessment process can also vary. In some accreditation programmes, the assessment is undertaken wholly by the accrediting organisation that developed the standards and manages the programme. This centralised approach enables the accrediting organisation to keep close control of the assessment process and the interpretation of the standards, but it can be expensive to do things this way. Other accreditation programmes focus more on setting the standards and leave the management of the assessment process much more to local organisations (which might be regional branches of a professional organisation, or regional health agencies) in collaboration with participants in the accreditation programme.

All accreditation programmes use assessors to undertake visits to the organisations being accredited, scrutinise the information provided, form an assessment of performance against the standards and produce a report. It is recognised that the role of the assessors in any accreditation programme is crucial, but the make-up of assessor teams, background of assessors, level of commitment to the role expected, training provided and arrangements for selecting assessors all vary from programme to programme.

In most cases, these assessors are drawn from professions involved in the organisation being accredited, and often a multidisciplinary team of assessors is used, involving, for example, a doctor, a nurse and a manager. Assessors usually fulfil the role on a very part-time basis, and hold substantive posts relevant to the organisations being accredited (for example, elsewhere in a similar organisation). A few accreditation programmes use full-time assessors, who then need to have substantial experience of the organisations being accredited before they take up their post as an assessor. In accreditation programmes that use only part-time assessors, a number of arrangements may be made to try to assure the quality of the accreditation process. Experienced assessors may be placed in charge of teams, while less experienced or new assessors assist or even just observe to begin with. A survey manager, working for the accrediting organisation may co-ordinate the assessment process and advise the assessors. Accreditation programmes usually offer some form of training for assessors, designed to help them develop the knowledge and skills needed to take on the role, and some impose selection requirements, only using as assessors those who have completed training successfully and who undertake a certain minimum number of assessments each year.

Presentation and dissemination of results

The results of the assessment process can be presented in a number of ways, both verbally (usually in an immediate feedback session at the end of an accreditation visit) and in writing (through a later and more formal report). Most fundamentally, the scoring of performance against the accreditation standards can be offered, so that the areas where standards were met or not met are identified. Often, this information is accompanied by a narrative commentary on performance, which highlights both particular areas for praise and commendation and areas where shortcomings or problems were found. In some accreditation programmes, a specific set of recommendations for action focused on the latter areas will be included. Finally, most accreditation programmes award some kind of quantitative score of performance, most commonly a dichotomous 'pass or fail' or some variant of this, although some also give a numeric measure of performance, such as the proportion of accreditation standards that were complied with.

In some accreditation programmes, the results of the accreditation process are entirely confidential to the organisation undertaking the accreditation, and may only be passed on to others with their consent. In other programmes, the overall result, and particularly the 'pass or fail' grade awarded, is made known to others, because it is used in decision making by healthcare funders or other agencies, and it may be made available to the general public. Further disclosure is rarer, but in some accreditation programmes all or most of the report on the organisation is made available to others, or even made public.

Impact and follow-up

One of the greatest unanswered questions about accreditation programmes is what impact they have on the organisations they accredit. There have been relatively few evaluations of accreditation programmes, and those that have taken place have often focused on describing the experience from the point of view of participants rather than objectively assessing the programme's impact. Once again, the impact should be assessed in the context of the purpose of the accreditation programme, and the likelihood of both intended and unintended impacts should be considered.

Most accreditation programmes attach some kind of time period or expiry to their recommendations and awards. Sustaining accreditation beyond that period requires the accredited organisation to resubmit itself for inspection at some point in the future. This means that most accreditation programmes have some form of follow-up incorporated into their design. However, periods of accreditation are frequently long – from 3 to 5 years – and so there can be an extended delay before the results and impact of the accreditation report are monitored. In some accreditation programmes, provision is made to pursue particularly important recommendations by undertaking a further visit, focused on the areas highlighted by the report, some months after the accreditation inspection.

Costs

The most obvious cost of any accreditation programme is the fee charged by the accrediting organisation to participants. Almost all accreditation programmes charge some sort of fee, either as a flat rate or based on some metric such as organisational size or financial turnover.

However, the fees charged by accreditation programmes rarely represent the true cost of running those programmes. First, much of the support needed to operate accreditation programmes is often obtained at no or little cost. For example, accreditation assessors often work for little or no fee, and their time is 'donated' by their employing organisation. Similarly, those involved in developing standards often take part in consultation exercises or committees with no recompense for the time and effort involved. In other words, there is a strong tradition of voluntarism in many accreditation programmes, reflecting their origins and ethos. Secondly, the organisations that run accreditation programmes are rarely commercial in nature, and are often wealthy professional or statutory agencies with other sources of income. They can, and do, cross-subsidise their accreditation programmes from other activities, either deliberately to encourage their development or inadvertently because they are not able to account for them separately. For these reasons, accreditation fees are a poor guide to real costs.

The other costs of the accreditation process fall on the organisation being accredited, and again these are usually subsumed into wider organisational costs rather than being specifically identified. Preparing for accreditation, providing the information that is required, and undertaking actions required to demonstrate compliance with the accreditation standards all involve costs in time and effort.

Box 2.2: A detailed framework for assessing accreditation programmes

Purpose
Is the primary objective quality improvement, informing decision making or accountability/ regulation?
Are the objectives clearly and explicitly stated?
How consistent are the stated objectives with each other, and what potential for conflict exists?

Participation and coverage
Is participation voluntary or mandatory?
If voluntary, what are incentives for participation, in terms of the benefits or rewards that it will bring, and what are the barriers that might deter participation?
If mandatory, what are the likely effects of forced participation on the programme?
What is the coverage of the programme?

Standards
At what level or stringency are the standards set – minimal, normative or optimal?
What is the content of the standards, in terms of their comprehensiveness, the areas covered, the approach to structuring or subdividing them, and their specificity?
How are the standards developed – what use is made of research evidence and of consensus development methods, how explicit, transparent and rigorous is the development process, what provision is there for the development of local variations, and is development likely to promote ownership?
How measurable are the standards – what guidance on assessment is offered, and what quantitative data are available to demonstrate adequate levels of validity and reliability?

continued

Assessment methods	What data sources (such as a written submission, special data collections, visits, etc.) are used in assessment? How much external involvement is there in the assessment? What is the make-up of the assessor team, from where are assessors drawn, and how are they selected and trained?
Presentation and dissemination of results	Is both verbal feedback and a written report provided? What does the report resulting from the accreditation review contain – detailed scoring against criteria, a narrative commentary on performance, specific recommendations for action or improvement, and an overall score or rating? Is the report confidential to the organisation being accredited, and who else might have access to the results, either in overview or in detail?
Impact and follow-up	What is known about the impacts – both intended and unintended – of the accreditation programme on participants? How is the accreditation process followed up, through subsequent visits or other mechanisms?
Costs	What are the fees or expenses charged to organisations to take part in the accreditation programme? What are the costs of the accreditation programme to the organisation which runs it, and how well are those costs known? What are the costs of taking part in the accreditation programme for organisations that participate, in areas such as the cost of preparation?

A framework for assessing accreditation programmes

The issues reviewed above are set out in summary in Box 2.2, which provides a detailed and structured framework with which accreditation programmes can be compared and contrasted. While there can be no objectively correct answers to the questions posed, the two criteria of internal consistency and contextual appropriateness discussed earlier provide an important test against which any accreditation programme should be tested.

Conclusions

It could be argued that the separate development of six accreditation programmes in primary care in the UK represents either healthy diversity, or unhelpful fragmentation. On the one hand, it may enable a number of different approaches to be piloted and tested, and important lessons may emerge from comparing these approaches (as the review in this chapter has already shown). Moreover, different accreditation programmes may be suited to different purposes. On the other hand, this level of fragmentation involves the development of separate sets of standards, assessment materials, assessor training courses and so on, and may cause some degree of confusion on the part of those working in primary care. In addition, such fragmentation may prevent any one accreditation programme from ever achieving the level of support and participation that would make it self-sustaining and widely recognised.

It would be a mistake to attempt to define the characteristics of a 'good' accreditation system, and then compare current or future accreditation programmes against that presumed benchmark, because so much depends upon the purpose to which the programme is to be put. Rather, the framework set out in this chapter can serve as a structure that makes it easier to compare and contrast different accreditation programmes and to see their similarities and differences. In the four following chapters, case studies of four different approaches to accreditation are presented and discussed, using the seven issues or dimensions identified in this framework.

1 Scrivens E (1996) A taxonomy of the dimensions of accreditation systems. *Social Policy and Administration.* **30**(2): 114–24.

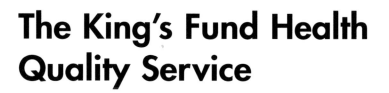

The King's Fund Health Quality Service

Andrew Corbett-Nolan

Introduction

The Health Quality Service (HQS) is an independent national organisation based at the King's Fund. It is engaged in creating programmes of accreditation for all sectors of healthcare provision, and in other initiatives relating to quality in healthcare, such as educational seminars and conferences, publications, benchmarking and comparative information, building on the work of the King's Fund Organisational Audit programme. The Health Quality Service is independent of both government and special interest and professional groups, and is the single largest healthcare accreditation provider in the United Kingdom. It has recently been recognised and accredited as a provider of accreditation itself by the United Kingdom Accreditation Service, an organisation relating to the Department of Trade and Industry which monitors and recognises certification bodies.

During 1998 and 1999 a great deal of development work has been going on at the Health Quality Service. A major set of enhancements has been developed for the programmes for NHS trusts and independent hospitals. A programme has been developed for hospices and another for nursing and residential care homes. Practical tools for engaging consumers are being developed. Educational programmes have been running since the summer of 1998, attracting large numbers of NHS participants. In primary care there have been several major initiatives, including two accreditation programmes, educational activities and an important publication for consumers.

Purpose of accreditation

Accreditation is an increasingly important tool for quality management and improvement in healthcare. In the United Kingdom there are a number of healthcare accreditation providers and, with the exception of the Health Quality Service they mainly operate programmes for particular services, professional groups or types of organisation. In the past few years most of the different accreditation providers have started exchanging information and collaborating. In 1998, the Health Quality Service initiated and sponsored the development of a collaborative group for UK healthcare accreditation organisations, the UK Accreditation Forum.

Taken together, accreditation initiatives dominate non-governmental efforts to improve quality in healthcare. For example, well over half of all NHS trusts have been involved with service or organisational accreditation work of one kind or another. Yet these accreditation activities have been applied mainly to secondary and tertiary care organisations and health services. Looking at the primary care accreditation work in the UK, coverage is much more limited. The King's Fund Health Quality Service has had a programme for primary healthcare teams for some years but it has been used by only around 250 practices – an important achievement but rather few, given the thousands of practices in the UK. Comparisons with the hospital accreditation programme, which has been taken up by 30% of NHS trusts and 50% of independent hospitals, are inevitable. Other accreditation initiatives in primary care have had a similarly limited take-up.

Participation and coverage

The low level of use of accreditation in primary care may seem strange in the light of its apparent advantages. Apart from the more obvious benefits to organisations of accreditation, such as increasing compliance with predetermined standards or the external recognition of quality, there are more practical considerations which one would imagine would be particularly to the point for smaller organisations such as general practices.

For example, many of the advantages of accreditation in healthcare have to do with the accreditation provider doing once what each client organisation would otherwise have to do itself. For example, the development of accreditation standards collects together all the national standards that apply to a particular type of organisation. These are then developed so that the implementation of the standards is clearly explained in the accreditation criteria and guidance. In other words, the accreditation agency collects together the various NHS circulars, health service guidance, legal requirements such as Health and Safety matters, as well as established examples of best practice and professional consensus. By doing this, the accreditation agency puts together at the core of its programme what would otherwise take each client organisation many hundreds of hours to do. Additionally, accreditation providers can do this better, having built up over time expertise in standards development and the kinds of linkages with organisations such as the medical Royal Colleges that no single healthcare providers could ever achieve.

Likewise, at the other end of the accreditation process is the assurance of the award itself. This can demonstrate to many different constituents what, in the absence of a reliable mark of quality, each would otherwise have to assess individually. Thus the accreditation programme acts as a proxy or intermediary for a number of stakeholders.

It seems that the small take-up in primary care accreditation to date has three causative factors. First, no accreditation provider has so far managed to produce a package for primary healthcare teams that is of an affordable price. HQS is a not-for-profit charitable organisation and its original primary care programme, on just a cost recovering basis, costs about £5 000 to each general practice in terms of the assessment fee alone. Although we would argue that general practices not going through the accreditation process may spend substantially more than this in time and other effort that could be avoided by using an accreditation programme, nevertheless the fee can be a real barrier to participation.

The fee charged for participating in the HQS primary care accreditation programme reflects its basic approach, which draws on that developed for NHS trusts, with each general practice having substantial support from HQS, training for staff, a peer review visit by a team of professionals and a full report commending innovation and excellence, confirming compliance with standards and providing recommendations for future development and service improvements. Some other accreditation schemes for primary care have also adopted this approach and, not surprisingly, have also found it expensive. For example, certification by an ISO 9000 accreditation agency might easily cost up to £15 000. Clearly, while the enthusiasts may be prepared to make this sort of level of investment in accreditation for their general practice, it stretches credibility to imagine a large-scale take-up at these cost levels. A radical rethink and a new approach are obviously needed, with the aim of developing a system that is much less resource demanding. To be successful, one would suggest that all schemes will have to contain their costs and aim at a much lower fee, although this should be done without compromises to the quality of the process.

Secondly, in the UK accreditation has not been well embedded in practice and, until recent years, has been something of a 'hobby' for a few enthusiasts. It has also been poorly understood. Commonly held perceptions of accreditation are often not that attractive, with concerns of a superficial 'tick box' check by inspectors against inventories of equipment, personnel and policy documents. The word itself draws the mind to the validation visit and an award certificate, rather than the process as a whole. It has taken large-scale educational efforts over a number of years by the accreditation providers to start to change this perception amongst the management of NHS trusts, and there is still a long way to go. It is hardly surprising, therefore, in the absence to date of substantial and sustained educational initiatives in the primary care sector on accreditation, that the argument has yet to be won that accreditation has a place to play.

Additionally, this poor understanding has not been helped by little support, and even some antipathy, from the establishment. This is now changing, and there have been early indications of support for accreditation from government and other important national organisations. The value of accreditation in terms of implementation of policy and delivering government aspirations is at long last being cautiously recognised.

The last factor explaining the poor take-up of accreditation in the primary care sector is that the climate of the healthcare market in the UK has been very dominated by concerns over cost and volume. However, recent initiatives from government are starting to change that. The government's consultation paper *A First Class Service: Quality in the New NHS* [1] set out a 10-year plan for the NHS, in which quality and performance issues will, in future, be central to healthcare decision making. The proposals focus initially on NHS trusts, though it has been made clear that the longer-term vision is that this new emphasis on quality will to all healthcare organisations apply in the coming years.

So, with the climate slowly but surely changing over time to favour accreditation, and educational initiatives gradually increasing the common understanding of the process, HQS believes that there will be a rapidly increasing use of accreditation in primary care in the future.

Standards for primary care groups

The government's White Paper, *The New NHS: Modern, Dependable,* [2] sets out an agenda for major change in the whole structure of healthcare in the UK. This continues the policy of a primary care led NHS, taking this concept one important further step forward with the creation of primary care groups and, in the future, primary care NHS trusts.

It has been no surprise that guidance on the setting up of primary care groups from the Department of Health has been developing slowly. However, the Department of Health commissioned the King's Fund Primary Care Programme and the Health Quality Service to develop and publish standards for primary care groups, and this work provides the promise of both a development agenda and an evaluation framework.

The style and approach of the Health Quality Service to standards development is to feed research and national guidance into multidisciplinary working groups, which then produce a draft for intensive national consultation. This draft can then be reviewed, field tested, revised and used as the basis for an accreditation programme. Health Quality Service standards are themselves reviewed and updated about every 2 years.

The first stages of the process have now been completed, and the Health Quality Service is now, in partnership with 15 UK commissioning authorities/boards, field testing the standards. In the meantime, and to be useful to those commissioning organisations now developing primary care groups, the standards that are being field tested have themselves been published.

These standards are quite basic, and as one would expect they address those matters which are of immediate concern to those setting up primary care groups. At this stage the focus is concerned with governance, management and organisation. The way Health Quality Service standards are expressed is that an overall standard is described, and then criteria for meeting this standard are stipulated, and guidance on what the criteria themselves mean in practice is then given where necessary. For primary care groups, the Health Quality Service has developed four standards, listed in Box 3.1.

Box 3.1: HQS standards for primary care groups

Standard 1: *The organisation of the primary care group.*

A constitution and organisational framework exists that enables the primary care group to meet its local, national and statutory responsibilities while remaining patient centred and accountable.

Standard 2: *Clinical governance*

There is an integrated and inclusive approach to clinical governance, which is supported at all levels of the primary care group, enabling continuous improvement of the quality of services and safeguarding high standards of care.

Standard 3: *The functions of the primary care group*

The primary care group acts in collaboration with others to improve the health of the population through the health improvement programme, develop primary and community services and commission secondary care.

Standard 4: *Development to higher levels*

The primary care group and its constituent parties assess, plan and develop its capacity to function at a higher level.

To demonstrate how the standards then relate to more detailed criteria, the clinical governance standard (standard 2 in Box 3.1) is organised into three sections:

- the framework for clinical governance
- quality
- clinical risk management.

Within the first section on the framework for clinical governance, there are 12 criteria focused on the lead clinicians for clinical governance within the primary care group as a whole, as well as the individual practices, and also addressing the clinical governance programme. As an example, criterion 2.6, which forms part of the consideration of the clinical governance programme is: 'The clinical governance programme is developed using local, multiprofessional expertise.'

The guidance to support this criterion suggests that this may be achieved through:

- local clinical audit groups
- academic institutions
- local clinical governance groups
- continuing professional development
- multiprofessional education and training
- evidence-based care
- organisational development expertise
- information and technology
- public health.

It cannot be emphasised too greatly that this work is the start of a long-term commitment to working with primary care groups over the coming years. These standards are the first draft, and will be built on and refined in the light of the field testing that takes place throughout 1999 and further guidance from central government as this emerges. It is likely, too, that as devolution develops, the differences between the health services in the four countries of the UK will increase rather than diminish, and that in time we will develop separate standards and programmes for primary care groups or their equivalents in Scotland, Wales and Northern Ireland.

With so much yet to be clarified about the future of primary care groups, the Health Quality Service has not endeavoured to make the standards rigorously measurable in this first instance. The current pilot programme will be looking at how different primary care groups put the structure and systems the standards describe into place, and at this stage being too prescriptive would not be helpful. Over time, when comparative information about primary care groups and compliance with standards and the certification aspect of accreditation become more important, rather than the developmental programme accreditation brings with it, then measurability and precision can be built into the programme. These are very first steps.

Standards for primary healthcare teams

The second primary care accreditation programme the Health Quality Service has been working on is aimed more at the primary healthcare teams themselves, and is taking forward the programme developed by King's Fund Organisational Audit over recent years.

At the practice level, a separate mechanism to the primary care group programme for quality improvement and assurance is needed. It is at this level that a great many accreditation providers have been doing work. Health Services Accreditation, for example, has been developing standards for primary healthcare teams looking at the organisation of the general practice, the delivery of effective clinical services and the commissioning of secondary care services by primary care organisations. Additionally, the Royal College of General Practitioners has developed its own scheme, described elsewhere in this book. Individual commissioning authorities and boards, such as South Essex Health Authority, have been operating accreditation schemes as ways of developing primary care capacity, distributing resources, rewarding innovation and excellence, and as a mechanism for performance management. As these responsibilities become the practical concerns of primary care groups rather than commissioning authorities and boards, the need for accreditation programmes targeted towards the primary healthcare team becomes more and more obvious.

The King's Fund Organisational Audit programme for primary healthcare teams has 17 separate standards, listed in Box 3.2.

Box 3.2: Standards for primary healthcare teams

1   The rights of all patients/clients and their carers, regardless of their age, disability, race gender or sexual orientation are recognised, respected and complied with by all staff involved in their care.

2   Staff are aware of, and respond to, the requirements of patients/clients with special needs (for example, the elderly and children).

3   There is a written mission statement, a philosophy and a set of objectives which act as a guide to planning, implementing and evaluating all aspects of the service.

4   There are written agreements/contracts for all healthcare provided by external agencies. These are monitoreed and reviewed regularly.

5   There are written signed agreements for all healthcare services provided by the facility.

6   The facility is organised, managed and staffed to provide safe, efficient and effective care to its patients/clients, to achieve its objectives, and to ensure high quality professional practice.

7   Continuing education and inservice programs are available to all staff to develop their knowledge and skills to meet the needs of the individual and the objectives of the service and the facility.

8   The primary healthcare team pursues excellence in all aspects of communication with colleagues, patients/clients, carers, health agencies and the local community. Confidentiality is maintained between staff and the patient/client, including information shared with relatives and/or carers.

9   The facility has appropriate and accurate information that is easily accessible to users and enables informed decisions to be made.

continued

10 There are written policies, procedures and protocols which reflect current knowledge and practice and are used to guide staff in their activities. They are the principles of good practice and are consistent with the objectives of the service and relevant regulations.

11 The facility provides a safe and healthy environment for patients/clients, staff and visitors.

12 Clinics are organised to provide specialised advice, support and services to a target population for specific, identified health needs.

13 Near patient testing conforms to protocols developed with an accredited pathology department. The monitoring of near patient testing is the responsibility of a designated senior medical laboratory scientific officer.

14 There are systems enabling patients/clients to gain access to services offered by the facility.

15 There is a systematic and individualised approach to patient/client care. Patients/clients receive treatment from appropriately trained staff.

16 The needs of patients/clients in the community are identified and the service required is delivered by the appropriate organisation.

17 The environment, facilities and equipment are maintained to a high standard which ensures the primary healthcare team achieves safe, efficient and effective care for all patients/clients.

18 The primary healthcare team ensures the provision of high quality care by its involvement in evaluation activities in line with the quality management plan and mission statement for the facility.

Assessment methods

The approach to developing primary care organisations to meeting these standards and implementing change and improvement was originally drawn from the model developed for NHS trusts. The Health Quality Service would provide a 'client manager' who acted as a contact point, provided ongoing support, co-ordinated a multidisciplinary peer-review assessment of the general practice and prepared the final accreditation. These client managers typically had a client portfolio of around a dozen organisations. A project manager from the general practice would be trained by the Health Quality Service, and this person would lead the accreditation process in the field. The practice would initially undertake a baseline audit to identify which standards were in place and which were not. This baseline audit would highlight the service development needs of the practice, and would be used to form a development plan for the practice to work on over the period of preparation for the survey, which might typically take around a year. A survey date would be arranged, and the Health Quality Service would put together a peer review team who themselves had been trained in both the Health Quality Service primary care programme and in assessment techniques. Leading up to the survey itself, the practice would prepare all the relevant documentation, which the client manager from the Health Quality Service would then come and examine. This all being in order, the survey would then go ahead to check compliance with the standards in practice, identify instances of best practice, innovation and excellence for commendation and identify items not up to standard which would need to be addressed in the future. The findings of the survey team would then be fed back to the practice at the end of the visit and written up in a report which would be sent to the practice afterwards. For the primary care programme, no accreditation certification was given, although the initial plan was to consider whether this would be useful in time.

This process was thorough and useful, but time consuming and expensive to provide. Bearing in mind the responsibilities of local commissioning organisations for developing primary care capacity, during 1997 the Health Quality Service worked with a number of commissioners to test out alternative ways of rolling the programme. The resulting concept, called the locally managed approach, was to essentially franchise local commissioning organisations to run the primary care programme for the practices in their area by cascade. The Health Quality Service would provide the standards to the commissioning organisation, and centrally train lead officers from health authorities and boards. These lead officers would then act as local client managers, supporting local practices through the process, training local peer-review surveyors, organising and running the visits, inspecting the documents and preparing the reports. The typical fee to a commissioning organisation for running the franchise over a 3-year period would be about £15 000 in the first year, and £5 000 in each of the second and third years. Divided amongst perhaps 75 practices the cost would be just several hundred pounds each – compared with about £5 000 per practice in the traditional approach.

The locally managed approach has been tested in several commissioning areas, and currently the results are being evaluated and a full-scale scheme for the UK is being finalised. However, with the development of primary care groups, the Health Quality Service believes that they, rather than commissioning authorities and boards, will have development and performance management responsibilities for primary care. In time, therefore, they may be the organisations running the locally managed approach.

More work is needed, though, on the primary healthcare team standards over the coming year, to feed into the locally managed approach over time. The original emphasis of the standards reflected the general approach of the Health Quality Service at the time they were developed. This approach has now moved on, and the emphasis has changed to success criteria for healthcare providers, and outputs as well as structures and processes.

Conclusions

In conclusion, the Health Quality Service is halfway through a development programme that will provide those developing and managing primary healthcare services with several useful mechanisms for improving and assuring quality. The Health Quality Service has looked at the environment in which primary care accreditation needs to be considered and has identified the critical success factors, these being: providing a service at a realistic price, educating the sector to understand the benefits of accreditation and providing mechanisms to help those charged with developing quality services in the NHS. Continued work aimed at influencing decision and policy makers in the four countries of the UK will remain very important.

The programme for primary care groups is currently being field tested and, at a practice level, work is well under way to roll out the locally managed approach. In future, it seems likely that accreditation will be much more widely used in primary care than it has been in the past.

1 Department of Health (1998) *A First Class Service: Quality in the New NHS*. The Stationery Office, London.
2 Department of Health (1997) *The New NHS: Modern, Dependable*. The Stationery Office, London.

4

The RCGP primary healthcare team-based practice accreditation programme

Theo Schofield and Clare Blakeway-Phillips

Introduction

The quality of care provided by any healthcare professional depends on their individual performance as well as the performance of the team and the system to which they belong. The Royal College of General Practitioners, as part of its quality network, set up a working party in 1994 to examine methods of assessing the performance of primary healthcare teams in practice, and to make recommendations to Council on the accreditation and re-accreditation of practices. Accreditation involves the external assessment of performance against agreed criteria. It can be used as a method of assuring the quality of the services that are being delivered, to identify areas requiring quality improvement, the need for resources, and to provide encouragement and support for professionals as their work and achievements are recognised. When the working party was convened the College did not have a policy, or sufficient evidence on which to base a policy, for the implementation of practice accreditation. We concluded, however, that there were good reasons for developing and evaluating methods that could be considered in future. The publication of the White Paper, *The New NHS: Modern, Dependable*, [1] with its emphasis on quality, proposals for clinical governance and the introduction of primary care groups, suggests that this view was correct.

The working party followed the College's recommended terminology that 'certification' refers to the individual, and 'accreditation' describes the assessment of the work of the primary healthcare team, and defined the 'team' as those people who identify themselves as working together to provide primary healthcare. The membership of the working group (set out in Box 4.1) was designed to reflect the disciplines and groups that had an interest in practice assessment, but the invitations were addressed to individuals rather than as representatives of any particular organisation.

Box 4.1: Membership of the RCGP Accreditation Working Party	
Theo Schofield	RCGP (convenor)
George Taylor	RCGP
Richard Hobbs	RCGP
Clare Blakeway-Phillips	Brent and Harrow Health Authority
Margaret Buttigieg	Health Visitors Association
Rosey Foster	Association of Managers in General Practice
Alan Torbet	Birmingham Family Health Services Authority
Laurence Buckman	General Medical Services Committee (GMSC)
Iona Heath	RCGP

The Royal College of General Practitioners had considerable experience of the assessment of doctors in their own practices, starting with *What Sort of Doctor?*, [2] the application of this method to the assessment of training practices,[3] and more recently Fellowship by Assessment.[4] The working group reviewed these methods, and also the work of the King's Fund Organisational Audit programme[5] (described in more detailed in Chapter 3), which has developed methods of assessing the organisation of primary care teams.

The conclusion from this review was that it should be possible to build on this experience to devise a method of assessment of the performance of the primary healthcare team that acknowledged their important values, that promoted the quality of their patient care and was feasible for, and acceptable to, any primary care team.

Purpose of team-based accreditation

The reasons for embarking on this enterprise included the following.

- Primary care is delivered by multidisciplinary teams, and while each member has their own professional responsibilities, the quality of the services they provide is dependent on the contribution of other team members.
- Previous programmes of practice-based assessment have all reported that involvement, both as assessors and as the assessed, has been educational, has increased professional satisfaction and has led to changes in practice.
- Patients should be assured that the services they are receiving are of a quality that meets their needs.
- Managers and purchasers need to know the range and quality of services that are being provided by those with whom they have contracts.
- Managers and professional groups concerned with the development of primary care need information on which to base the allocation of resources.

We therefore believed that it was timely to conduct a project to develop and evaluate practice accreditation to inform future policy.

The working party discussed the principles that they believed should guide the development of accreditation in primary healthcare. We wished to adhere to the principle of professional self-regulation for all members of the team, because we believed it was more likely to be acceptable and effective at promoting change and development.

- The underlying ethos of accreditation should be to support quality improvement in practice, and to be closely related to practice development and education.
- In the first instance, any method of accreditation should be voluntary, but designed so that every practice could take part.
- Accreditation should be concerned with the practice team and its functioning, and the services the team provide.
- The criteria for accreditation should reflect the needs and views of patients.
- Assessments should be by professional peers, and therefore multidisciplinary.
- Assessment methods should build on existing methods of performance review in practice.
- The method of assessment must be demonstrably valid and reliable.
- The process of accreditation should be locally owned.
- The response to underperformance should be supportive and remedial.

Standards

The working party drew up a set of criteria for the services provided by the team, and the way the team functioned. The draft criteria were drawn from a variety of sources, including the documentation used by the previous approaches to practice accreditation described above, as well as the Terms and Conditions of Service for Doctors in General Practice. We believed that, wherever possible, criteria should not just reflect professional or patient opinion, but also be based on evidence of a relationship to outcomes. However, such evidence was frequently unavailable.

It was our intention that the standards should be broad statements of principle, while the criteria were specific statements that should be assessable. However, we included some statements that were regarded as important and amenable to judgement and discussion, for example the health of team members, but which were not measurable. Levels of performance should not just define minimum standards, but indicate markers to encourage progress in practice. They were therefore divided into those that were essential, normal good practice and desirable. This was done by the local steering group to take account of variations in local circumstances. Essential criteria were those that related to terms and condition of service, professional requirements, legal requirements or safety of practice. The standards are summarised in Table 4.1, and set out in full in the appendix.

Table 4.1: Summary of RCGP standards

Services for patients	The primary care team
Accessibility	Team values
Communication	Training and continued learning
Prescribing	Teamworking
Investigations	Records
Preventive care and health promotion	Management
Chronic disease care	Quality assurance and audit
Children's health	Premises
Maternity services	
Continued care at home	
Family planning and women's health	
Mental health services	
Elderly surveillance	
Minor operations	

Methods of assessment

The method of assessment that was developed was similar to those used in other programmes, but the volume of preparation and documentation was kept to a minimum to make it more feasible for all teams to take part. The stages in the process were as follows.

1 The team was visited to give them the criteria and to explain what was required.
2 The team assessed themselves against these criteria and prepared for the assessment.
3 The team prepared a brief practice profile and assembled their existing documentation, e.g. their brochure and any protocols, procedures or audits that they have.
4 A questionnaire, designed by the College of Health, was sent to a sample of the practice's patients, and the responses were collated by the facilitator.
5 The visiting team, a GP, a practice or community nurse and a practice manager, were sent the documentation and planned their visit.
6 The assessors visited the practice for a day, observed its working, interviewed team members and reviewed a sample of records, using a structured grid that relates sources of information to the criteria that are assessed.
7 Feedback was given, initially verbally at the end of the day, and then in a written report, that described the team's achievements, identified areas for improvement and made recommendations for future development.
8 The local group considered the report, and accredited the team.

Piloting the programme in Brent and Harrow

The working party invited faculties of the College to express interest in developing and conducting a pilot of these proposals. Replies were received from five faculties, and one faculty, North-West Thames, was able to obtain funding for a pilot to be conducted in collaboration with Brent and Harrow Health Authority. This was led by Dr Mahendra Mashru, Chairman of the Faculty Board, and Clare Blakeway Phillips, Head of Quality and Professional Development in the health authority, who was able to provide substantial support both to the steering group and to the participating practices during the project.

A multidisciplinary steering group was set up to develop the project with the remit of:

- reviewing the draft criteria and proposals for the method of assessment, to ensure that they were acceptable and reflected local concerns
- identifying 12 practice teams willing to take part in the pilot
- training the visiting assessors
- managing the practice assessments
- reviewing the results and drawing conclusions about the future development of team-based accreditation.

This group contained representatives of the faculty, Medical Audit Advisory Group, community health council, GP tutors, health authority and practice and community nurses. This group was essential to create local ownership for the project, to ensure that the criteria met local concerns, including those of patients, and, most importantly, to mobilise educational resources to support practices through the accreditation process.

Once the practice teams had agreed to participate in the pilot they were given the criteria and guidelines on the assessment process. The degree of preparation that the teams chose to undertake varied from a single team member completing the assessment forms and arranging the assessment visit, 'Take us as you find us', to other teams who used it as an opportunity for the whole team to review themselves against the criteria and for teambuilding.

The practices were asked to nominate people from their team to be trained as assessors. Twenty people – GPs, nurses and practice managers – volunteered and attended a training day to become familiar with the criteria, to help them plan their assessment visits and to practise appropriate skills. These included interviewing, listening, observation, giving feedback and report writing. The assumption that all health professionals would have these skills had already led to insufficient time being provided for assessor selection and training.

A team of three assessors, a GP, nurse and practice manager, was assigned to each practice, and they agreed the timetable for their visit with the practice. They ensured that as many members of the team would be interviewed as possible, and that time would be allowed for observing the reception area and reviewing the records and documentation. At the end of the day the assessors gave brief verbal feedback, which was an opportunity to check the accuracy, and to some extent the acceptability, of their conclusions to the team. The team then prepared a written report detailing the strengths of the team and making recommendations for future development. Both parts of the feedback required sensitivity and skill, as well as experience of primary care on which to base recommendations.

The written reports could be used by the team as a basis for their practice and personal development plans. Three-quarters of the recommendations were accepted by the practices, and of these 60% had resulted in action within 6 months of the assessment. The local steering group also reviewed the reports and gave accreditation certificates to the teams who met all the essential criteria. Nine practices were accredited while three were asked to take steps to fulfil some essential criteria before being accredited.

The local steering group was also able to consider whether any common themes came out of the assessments, and to provide help to remedy them. Courses were provided on the use of practice computers, on needs assessment, and user and community involvement. These were open to all practices in the district. The teams who were involved also reported the value of visiting other practices, learning from them and developing a greater sense of collegiality between practices in the area.

Impact and follow-up

Once the pilot phase was completed, a meeting was held with Brent and Harrow practices to share the results of the evaluation and to discuss the way forward locally. Those who had participated in the pilot felt strongly that other practices should be able to benefit from participation as they had done. They also felt that they did not want to lose the skills they had gained as assessors. New practices expressed interest in participating. One of the most valuable contributions to the meeting was from a single-handed GP, who encouraged her colleagues, especially the single-handed GPs and small practices, by saying that they should participate because if she could successfully undertake the process, they could as well. Through her encouragement, a single-handed GP and some small practices, who do not normally put themselves forward for new schemes, did so.

With the development of primary care groups, the practices were encouraged to think how an accreditation scheme such as this could provide a framework for their clinical governance arrangements. Staff within the primary care group could be trained in co-ordinating the scheme. It could also be adapted to suit their primary care groups' needs and local action plans could be incorporated, for example management of diabetes. Peer review would enable the practices to learn from each other, as well as ensuring that agreed ways of working were in place.

The RCGP Accreditation Working Party agreed to continue to oversee the programme and nine further practices signed up to participate. More expressed interest, but due to personal pressures or pressures of primary care group development, asked to defer to the following year. The next wave of practices were asked to review the criteria but they suggested no changes.

Six more assessors were trained (four from these practices and two from the Community Trust). This time a selection procedure was introduced and, after the training, it was agreed that four of them would act as assessors as the other two felt unconfident in the role. Instead of extending the training, we agreed that there should be guidance and feedback on the assessment visits by either the co-ordinator or more experienced assessors.

Now that primary care groups (PCGs) are in place, some practices are beginning to see the potential for accreditation and how it could help them develop practices within their PCG, especially in bringing them up to a 'level playing field'.

Costs

The costs of the pilot programme included the following.

- The cost of the time spent by the practices in preparing for and participating in the assessment. This was not reimbursed, and the teams who volunteered said that they were willing to do this in return for receiving an external assessment.
- The time of the visiting assessors. All the assessors were paid locum costs to cover their absence, and time for preparation and report writing.
- Local co-ordination of the programme. The major cost of the programme was the time of the local co-ordinator for convening the local group, visiting practices and supporting their preparation, training assessors, arranging visits and supervising the writing of reports. This not only required time but also a considerable level of expertise.

The cost of assessing each practice includes the marginal cost of the visit and the contribution to the fixed costs, which depends on the number of practices involved. We estimate that the total cost would be between £1000 and £2000 per practice.

Conclusions

The external evaluation of this pilot programme of accreditation is described in Chapter 7. We believe that this approach achieved our aims, which were to devise a method of assessment of the work of primary care teams that was rigorous and also supportive and educational, that promoted quality and team development, and could be delivered locally to all primary care teams. The RCGP has now convened a new multidisciplinary group to take this work forward in the context of the new NHS and clinical governance.[6]

Acknowledgements

The success of this development so far has depended on the efforts of the working party, the local Steering Group, the local co-ordinator, and above all the practices that took part in the pilot. The support we have received from The Royal College of General Practitioners, its North-West Thames Faculty and from Brent and Harrow Health Authority has also been essential. We are grateful to them all.

1 Department of Health (1997) *The New NHS: Modern, Dependable*. The Stationery Office, London.

2 Royal College of General Practitioners (1985) *What Sort of Doctor?* Report from General Practice 23. Royal College of General Practitioners, London.

3 Schofield TPC and Hasler JC (1984) Approval of trainers and training practices in the Oxford Region. *BMJ.* **288:** 538–40, 612–14, 688–9.

4 Royal College of General Practitioners (1990) *Fellowship by Assessment*. Occasional Paper 50. Royal College of General Practitioners, London.

5 Blakeway-Phillips C (1993) *Report on the King's Fund Organisational Audit Primary Care Project.* King's Fund, London.

6 Department of Health (1998) *A First Class Service: Quality in the New NHS*. The Stationery Office, London.

5

Practice accreditation: the Northumberland approach

Ann Foreman and Peter Mitford

Introduction

This chapter examines the experience and results that can be drawn from the Northumberland accreditation programme and ways in which accreditation can be strengthened at a local level.

In 1993, the General Medical Services Committee (GMSC) of the British Medical Association produced a discussion paper on practice accreditation/re-accreditation. As is usual when accreditation is considered, concern was expressed about whether such a tool would be used as a vehicle for quality improvement or as a method of policing and regulating primary care.[1] It was clear at that time that the GMSC was not ready to endorse accreditation, but many appreciated the value of such a tool and could foresee that at some stage primary care professionals and organisations would be held to account for the quality of care they provided. One member of the GMSC, Dr Graham Ridley (now

Northumberland Local Medical Committee (LMC) chairman) returned to Northumberland from the debate convinced that a simple system of accreditation, devised, owned and applied locally, would be a powerful stimulus to quality development and a way of helping practices overcome their fears and suspicions of this approach.

Northumberland Family Health Services Authority (later Northumberland Health Authority) was then in the early stages of involvement with the King's Fund Organisational Audit and Investors in People. These and other important developmental tools, notably RCGP Fellowship by Assessment, have since been encouraged and supported in all interested practices.[2] They represent major undertakings and inevitably focus on more advanced practices. However, it was clear at an early stage that a simple and more universally applicable tool was desirable.

Discussion between Northumberland Local Medical Committee and the health authority ultimately led to an agreement to develop a local system of practice accreditation, and a steering group with membership drawn from the LMC and health authority was established.

Purpose of local accreditation

The steering group decided to adopt a modular approach to ensure that the increased workload resulting from the process of measuring against selected standards was contained at a level with which practices could cope. It was agreed that, to make the tool relevant to all practices, the lowest level of each standard should potentially be achievable by all. The first module developed by the steering group concentrated on practice organisation rather than clinical issues, but it was agreed that clinical performance would be part of subsequent modules when practices were more comfortable with the approach.

The stated aim of the first module of local practice accreditation was to improve the organisation of primary healthcare teams and enable them to deliver a better level of patient care.

The following main objectives were identified.

- To compare organisational performance against standards. Primary healthcare teams are small businesses, which have evolved over time. Most are managed (or, more accurately, administered) by individuals who have learned by doing rather than having any formal training as managers. Systems and processes often reflect what has always been done, and are characterised by locally devised and sometimes unconventional solutions to common problems. Many practices still operate in considerable isolation and have no yardsticks by which to judge their own performance. Objective standards can provide a 'safe' introduction to performance assessment without the risks of exposure for poor performance and the defensive behaviour that is likely to engender.
- To improve practice organisation. Accreditation indicates the areas in which current practice organisation falls short of the ideal, and provides the foundation for an action plan to develop or improve organisation in those areas.
- To establish guidelines and protocols. Working to simple guidelines or protocols ensures consistency in practice and provides new or inexperienced members of staff with a point of reference from which to work. The organisational standards help in the development of guidelines and protocols.
- To demonstrate commitment to quality. By taking part in the local practice accreditation programme, practices were demonstrating their own commitment to quality improvement.
- To identify and share good practice. Good practice exists in primary care, often in the most unexpected places. Its existence is often unknown and it is frequently not shared with others. Accreditation facilitates the identification of examples of good practice and helps with dissemination through networking, mentoring and so on.
- To promote educational development. It is still the case that much educational activity in primary care is not focused on clearly identified learning or development needs. Accreditation allows the precise identification of educational needs of staff and so facilitates the development of educational programmes to meet those needs.

It was agreed that local practice accreditation should be part of a drive to ensure continuous quality improvement and should not be used to make a simplistic pass or fail assessment. The health authority was committed to resourcing educational needs that emerged from the exercise and gave guarantees that the outcomes would not be used as a policing exercise.

Participation and coverage

At the time of the local practice accreditation exercise there were 52 general practices in Northumberland. The vast majority, 50 practices, completed their own self-assessment against the accreditation standards. Only two practices did not take part – one refused and another was in the process of dissolution at the time. This high level of participation was achieved even though the accreditation process was entirely voluntary.

Following the self-assessment by practices, arrangements were made to verify the results externally, through an assessor visiting each practice. Some practices already had some experience of this form of external verification – 12 had taken part in the King's Fund Organisational Audit programme for primary care – and so it was not thought necessary to visit them. Of the remainder, 37 agreed to undergo external verification and only one practice refused.

Overall, 49 out of 52 practices (94%) completed the whole process of self-assessment and external verification.

The standards

The standards were derived and piloted during 1995 and distributed to all practices in Northumberland in May 1996. The standards selected for inclusion in the first module were:

- access to surgery consultation
- patient's complaints procedure
- handling and storage of records
- team meetings
- records management.

A small multidisciplinary group drawn from primary care teams, the health authority and the Community Trust devised the standards. They were structured into a number of levels so that practices could be graded at the appropriate level and, as the same standards were set for all practices, comparative assessment of performance was possible. The standards were then piloted, first by circulating them widely for comments and then by testing them in four practices. The standards are summarised in Box 5.1.

Box 5.1: Standards used in the Northumberland local practice accreditation programme

1 Access to surgery consultation

The practice appointment system should offer a degree of flexibility to ensure easy access for patients.

Level 1   The practice has an appointments system.
Level 2   The practice has a system whereby any patient can be seen if requested the same day.
Level 3   The practice has a system for seeing extra patients.
Level 4   The practice has a system for monitoring the availability of appointments.

2 Patients' complaints procedure

The practice has an in-house complaints procedure, which is used positively to raise quality standards.

Level 1   The practice has a system in place for dealing with complaints.
Level 2   The practice has a protocol for complaints.
Level 3   The practice has a method for recording complaints and their response to them.
Level 4   The practice reviews complaints regularly and takes action accordingly.

continued

3 Handling and storage of results

The practice has an effective system that ensures that all results are seen by a clinically competent person and abnormal results are followed up.

Level 1   The practice has a system in place to ensure that all reports are seen by a clinically competent person.

Level 2   The practice has a system to follow up abnormal reports, ensuring action is taken.

Level 3   The results are stored so that enquiries can be answered quickly and efficiently.

Level 4   There is a protocol in place for informing patients of their results.

Level 5   Results can be retrieved for research and audit purposes.

4 Team meetings

There is evidence of regular, multidisciplinary meetings for the primary healthcare team (PHCT); this would include representation from each discipline, with a formal agenda and minutes, including action points.

Level 1   The practice holds a partners' meeting.

Level 2   The practice holds meetings between partners and the practice manager.

Level 3   The practice holds meetings between the partners and clinical and administrative staff.

Level 4   The practice holds meetings of the PHCT, including community staff.

5 Patient records management

The practice has appropriate and accurate information that is easily accessible to staff and enables informed decisions to be made.

Level 1   The practice records basic identification data for all patients.

Level 2   The practice records further identification data for all patients.

Level 3   The practice has efficient systems (manual or computerised) for recording and filing clinical data.

Level 4   The practice uses alert markers (manual or computerised) on the records of patients with similar names, hypersensitivities or chronic diseases.

The assessment method

Each practice received an assessment booklet, containing an introduction, an explanation of how to complete it, an outline of each standard and a self-assessment sheet for each standard for them to complete. The assessment booklet was accompanied by a letter from the secretary of the local medical committee and the director of primary care development at the health authority, endorsing the approach and expressing the hope that all practices would participate. Practices were asked to complete the self-assessment and return it to the clinical audit development manager at the health authority.

The credibility of practice self-assessments was ensured by providing a mechanism for externally verifying the results, to check that practices had followed the guidance in the assessment booklet and to make a direct examination of supporting evidence. External verification visits to practices were undertaken by two staff who had experience in acting as surveyors for the King's Fund Organisational Audit programme in primary care. The verification visit was preceded by a letter to the practice manager outlining what was expected and requesting access to the following information:

- a copy of the surgery appointments book
- a copy of the practices' complaints procedure
- a formal protocol for handling results
- evidence of agendas and minutes from practice meetings
- a number of sets of medical records selected at random.

Overall, the verification process proved successful. Discussions with the practices were most fruitful when both practice manager and GPs were present. Future modules will require the involvement of other disciplines.

Presentation and dissemination of results

The results of the local practice accreditation programme were collated and disseminated to all practices in April 1997. Quantitative analysis demonstrated a significant level of achievement across the county, though some areas of non-compliance were highlighted as potential areas for development and formed the basis for a practice action plan. A series of graphs showing levels of compliance with the standards set out in Box 5.1 are shown in Figure 5.1. Qualitative information was presented that had been gathered throughout the external verification process, in which practice managers and general practitioners had time to reflect upon and discuss the problems they faced in a non-threatening environment. This qualitative information proved to be particularly important in understanding the development needs of the practice.

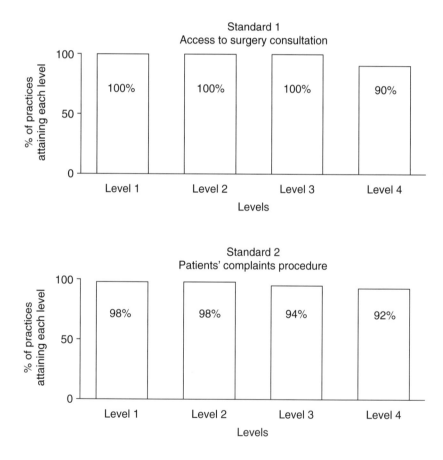

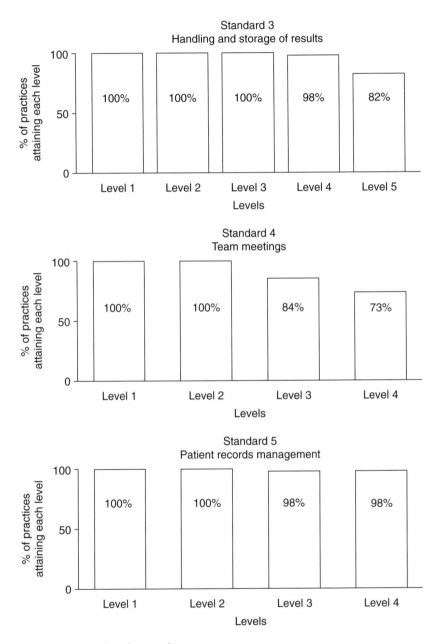

Figure 5.1 Levels of compliance.

Three important lessons emerge from the use of the results of the programme in Northumberland. First, the identification and commendation of good practice by trained external assessors, independent of the practice, has a powerful positive effect on team morale, provides recognition of achievements and can be a stimulus for future efforts. Secondly, when potential areas for improvement were identified, non-judgemental feedback in the form of recommendations for improvements was given, and practices responded very positively to this and were happy to agree to subsequent re-accreditation to show that improvements had indeed taken place. Thirdly, accreditation should not be introduced at all if the development, education and training needs it highlights are not going to be addressed subsequently. Available resources usually dictate that they will not all be addressed immediately, but practices will accept a plan to deliver over an agreed time scale.

Impact of accreditation

The main achievement of the local practice accreditation programme in Northumberland was the production of a simple set of measurable standards that primary care teams found credible, understandable and relevant, and the subsequent willing involvement of such a large percentage of practices in assessment against those standards.

The standards were deliberately set at an achievable level, and changes were demonstrated in a number of areas. Staff commitment to the process was engendered or strengthened through positive feedback and recognition of their needs. The team effort involved in preparing for accreditation helped to promote teamworking. The approach helped to spread consistently good practice across teams, through networking and other mechanisms, and to identify future training, development and other needs in a systematic way.

The accreditation programme identified many support needs in practices that we had not anticipated, and the level of need outstripped our ability to provide support. This was an important lesson learned and we will be better prepared for the outcomes of the second module.

Qualitative feedback from practice managers indicated a high level of anxiety about their role and its development. To address this a management competencies programme was established, based upon Management Charter Institute (MCI) standards at levels 4 and 5. The course was provided using experienced managers from primary care development and general practice, and the National Vocational Qualification (NVQ) that it resulted in has been externally accredited by the University of Northumbria Business School. It has been specially designed to address the needs of existing practice managers and those employed by practices who might reasonably aspire to such a role.

Informal discussions with practices indicated that they would value help in identifying future development needs, relating current progress to areas of agreed good practice, and identifying areas where teams require help. This resulted in the development of a self-assessment tool kit, which covers five key development areas:

- service development
- team development
- finance
- information management
- public involvement.

The tool kit has been used, extensively in whole or part. At the time of writing, eight teams are making use of it.

Next steps in local practice accreditation

The second module of local practice accreditation in Northumberland is soon to be launched. The new standards are based upon areas identified as relevant by primary healthcare teams during the verification and evaluation of the first module:

- health and safety
- staff appraisal
- training development planning
- chronic disease management
- prescribing.

The successful external assessment, which proved so valuable, will remain, with the addition of a general practitioner to the verification process. The verifiers will also revisit the practice reports from the first module, giving primary healthcare teams the opportunity to discuss their previous results and action plans, with a view to being re-accredited at a higher level.

The modules and the process are cyclical and we are therefore continually building up a picture of the activity and quality of primary care services in Northumberland. This allows us to refocus and respond actively to the training and development needs of teams from the evidence of practice accreditation data.

Costs

The local practice accreditation programme in Northumberland has not been individually costed. Both the local medical committee and the health authority consider it to be a high priority and therefore justifiably a core component of the roles of the staff involved in developing and implementing the programme.

To demonstrate its commitment, the local medical committee contributed £3 000 to pump prime the process, and GPs and others involved in developing the standards gave their time free. Involvement was free to participant practices. An estimate of the costs of the programme (excluding costs incurred by individual practices in, for example, preparing for accreditation) is given in Table 5.1. It includes the costs of time for health authority staff and general practitioners, travel expenses, printing and distribution, etc.

Table 5.1: Costs of local practice accreditation in Northumberland

Procedure	Cost (£)
Preparation of the standards	4 000
Analysis of self-assessment data and production of reports	2 500
External verification process – visits to practices	3 000
Final report and feedback	2 000
Total cost	11 500
Cost per practice	235

It should be borne in mind that the development costs arising from implementing the recommendations and ideas for improvement that emerged from accreditation were significant. For example, the self-assessment tool kit cost about £10 000 to develop, and the management competencies programme cost around £40 000 to provide. All other development support needs were provided from within the existing resources of the primary care audit group, the primary care development directorate of Northumberland Health Authority, and the Northumberland Community Health NHS Trust (now Northumbria Healthcare NHS Trust).

Conclusions

Practice accreditation can be a challenging experience for primary healthcare teams,[3] and opening their doors to external review can be difficult, but our experience convinces us that participation in the accreditation process strengthens and empowers practices. Having the motivation and the ability to look critically at your own performance, to acknowledge where there are problems or room for improvement, and to address your own development needs is an indication of professional maturity.

Local practice accreditation delivers a solid foundation upon which to build the broader quality agenda, but it may have wider potential uses, such as a common quality management and improvement mechanisms for primary care groups as part of their arrangements for clinical governance. Increasingly, as general practitioners face rising levels of litigation for clinical negligence, accreditation may be a tool for controlling risk and reducing the incidence of adverse events. In the future, we may see participation in accreditation being rewarded through the payments system for general practice, replacing some of the rather outdated payment mechanisms contained in the current contract with some that recognise the important of quality improvement in primary care.

1 Scrivens E (ed) (1995) *Issues in Accreditation*. Working papers 1–6. Keele University Press, Keele.

2 Scrivens E (1998) Widening the scope of accreditation – issues and challenges in community and primary care. *International Journal for Quality in Healthcare.* 10(3): 1991–7.

3 Sheehan M Doolan T and Veitch C (1996) Application of primary healthcare standards to a developing community health group: a rural case history. *Australian and New Zealand Journal of Public Health.* 20(2): 201-9.

6

Training practice accreditation

John Hasler

Introduction

The history of general practitioner training in the United Kingdom goes back to the beginning of the National Health Service. At the outset, provision was made for general practitioners to have young doctors (known as trainees) attached to them for the purposes of learning about family medicine. Payment was made to the general practitioner for the supervision and for reimbursement of the trainee's salary and other expenses. The scheme was not widely taken up during the 1950s and early 1960s, partly because of the decline in morale generally in primary medical care and partly because the trainee often received little or no teaching. The trainer appointments were made by local medical committees until the responsibility for the arrangements were taken over by regional general practice education committees in 1973.

During the late 1960s and early 1970s, interest in making the trainee scheme more educational increased, stimulated by developments in GP education in Wessex and elsewhere. With an educational, as opposed to a political, body assuming responsibility for trainer appointments, the scheme started to change from a mere attachment to a proper educational programme. This period in a GP's development, which was limited to 12 months, was (and largely still is) the only time actually spent in general practice, the remainder usually being spent entirely in junior hospital posts. Although it is the trainer who is appointed, because of the importance of the learning environment and the contribution of other professionals, over the years the practice has come under increasing scrutiny. It is now generally accepted that however good the trainer, if the practice is inadequate in some way, an appointment cannot be made. Nevertheless, the fact that it is the GP personally who is appointed creates potential problems now, at a time when the importance of the team is being stressed.

Purpose

The purpose, then, of trainer and training practice appointments is to ensure that a young doctor is reasonably prepared and equipped to work in general practice. However, it is now generally recognised that with the increasing sophistication of primary healthcare, the trainee year is insufficient to provide all that is required, and it therefore forms a basis on which further development can take place.

The primary purpose of appointing trainers is to make a pass or fail judgement. But what all trainers and their practices need is an assessment procedure that gives them detailed feedback on their strengths and development points. Since, in the vast majority of cases, the trainer is not being failed, it is perfectly possible to achieve this second aim as well. Nevertheless, it must be said that, although this was the approach adopted in Oxford in the early 1980s, it was not what occurred in all parts of the country. Many people felt that the two aims could not be combined. Equally, many of the assessments were not long or comprehensive enough to allow a detailed development feedback. Moreover, the problem was often made worse by the fact that in some regions the assessment reports were not seen by the trainers themselves.

Participation and coverage

Regional GP education committees were set up in the early 1970s as subcommittees of the regional medical postgraduate committees, although in relation to trainer appointments they are autonomous. At the same time, regional advisers in general practice (now known as directors of postgraduate general practice education) were appointed on a sessional basis, and became the executive officers of the GP committees. Criteria and standards and the method of appointment and re-appointment were established in each region, and interest in the scheme rose. By the 1990s around 10% of all GPs were appointed as trainers and, since the vast majority were in partnerships, around a quarter of all practices were training practices.

For the duration of the 1970s GP training remained voluntary, but after much discussion it was made mandatory in 1981 and shortly afterwards a further 2 years of hospital training (or the equivalent) were also made compulsory for anyone wishing to become a principal in general practice. Training is now required for any doctor working in general practice, regardless of position. By the late 1980s general practice had become so popular as a career that multiple applications for training places were being made, and it was relatively unusual for a training practice not to have a trainee.[1] That situation has now changed and, with demand falling, it is not unusual for training practices to have no trainee (or registrar, as trainees are now known).

Standards

National developments

With the advent of regional educational bodies, attention began to be directed to the criteria and standards that should be expected of trainers and their practices.

A national committee – the Joint Committee on Postgraduate Training for General Practice (JCPTGP) – was set up in the mid-1970s to oversee the activities of regional GP education committees. The

JCPTGP itself promulgated a number of mandatory standards, largely related to such matters as medical records.[2] But the Joint Committee was never able to identify criteria and standards in any detail, partly because of its national remit and partly because of tensions in the committee between ardent educationalists and pragmatic medico-politicians who made up the bulk of the membership. It was therefore left to the regions to set out the expectations in detail. In 1998 the JCPTGP itself assumed responsibility for appointing the training practices, although in practice the regional committees still deal with day-to-day appointments.

Indeed, the difficulties for any national body to set and police detailed standards are well exemplified by the situation the JCPTGP finds itself in. Since the situation regarding all developments relating to standards in medical care is a dynamic one, it is virtually impossible to set out criteria and standards that both stimulate progressive practices and are fair to less developed ones (see later).

The JCPTGP carries out inspection visits of its own to training practices in all regions, to check on the standards being operated by regional committees. Because the JCPTGP is now ultimately responsible for practice appointments, it can, if it so wishes, remove approval as a result of one of these visits.

Regional development

Inevitably, the regional committees varied (and still do vary) in what they demanded of the practices within their geographical remit. The challenges facing primary care are different in different places, and therefore what can realistically be expected of practices working in areas with a high turnover of patients, large-scale deprivation and high average list sizes is less than what might be expected elsewhere. Another very important factor is the leadership demonstrated by the Director of Postgraduate GP Education, and some directors have achieved more than others.

A good example of the need for flexibility over criteria and standards is out-of-hours care. In the 1970s, most regions expected training practices and their trainees to do their own out-of-hours cover within an internal practice rota or in one with a neighbouring practice. Gradually arrangements changed, with large urban areas starting to use deputising services. In regions where the use of deputising services became widespread, it was unrealistic to continue to apply the original criteria on out-of-hours care to training practices. By the late 1980s and early 1990s, regions were applying different criteria, depending on their local circumstances. With the advent of widespread co-operatives in the mid-1990s, criteria had to be modified again.

Criteria and standards

It is helpful to draw a distinction between criteria and standards. Criteria indicate in what areas targets are expected to be achieved. An example might be (and often was) 'All medical records should contain an up-to-date summary sheet'. Standards, on the other hand, indicate the level of performance that is desirable or acceptable at any particular time. It also sometimes implies uniformity and so 'level of performance' may be a better set of words. In relation to the previous example, the standard or level of performance might be that in a certain year '80% of medical records must be summarised'. In fact, what is important is movement. At the end of the 1990s, some practices have been training for much longer than others and it would be unfair to expect a new practice to achieve everything that a long-established training practice has. The fact that some of them do, says more about some established practices than it does about new ones. What GP committees and directors look for, if they are wise, is continuing development rather than static standards. This avoids the danger that complacency may be produced by achieving minimum levels of performance.

Setting the standards

Any system of standard setting by other people is potentially difficult. Individuals often resent what is seen as imposition of criteria and standards, especially when these have implications for income and status. In the early days, when the existing training practices had frequently been used to only minimal appointment hurdles, it was particularly so. GP committees and regional advisers moved carefully, some more so than others. But periodically, over the years, regions have decided that a major review of criteria and standards was needed and new requirements have been drawn up.

Such a time occurred in Oxford in the early 1980s. By then it was clear that a review was needed and this had been stimulated by the development of work on consultation in general practice proceeding in Oxford at that time.[3] The regional adviser and his colleagues recognised that in order for the new proposals to work they would need to be acceptable to the majority of trainers, and that had to be taken into account when deciding on the new arrangements.

The method and list of criteria has been described in full elsewhere:[4] they remain broadly the same 15 years later, although the standards and expectations have risen. A regional working party was established with representatives of all the trainers, together with trainees, GP vocational training course organisers and the regional adviser and his associate adviser. The working party was asked to draw up draft criteria, which were then circulated for comment before a final version was produced. It drew heavily, both for criteria and methodology, on work done previously by the Royal College of General Practitioners.[5]

The criteria are prefaced by a statement of principle, describing briefly what they cover, followed by a section relating to the trainer, then the practice and finally the teaching itself. The original criteria were grouped under a number of headings, which still remain largely the same today:

The trainer: professional values
previous experience
clinical competence
continuing education
commitment to teaching
preparation for teaching
teaching ability
contribution to the local training scheme
membership of the RCGP

The practice: partnership responsibilities
                 time for teaching and other educational activities
                 list size and workload
                 arrangements for seeing patients
                 night and weekend work
                 medical records
                 preventive medicine
                 performance review
                 premises
                 libraries and journals
                 staff, equipment and organisation
                 healthcare team
                 practice meetings
                 contract of employment
Teaching: assessment and curriculum planning
                 teaching methods

It is important to stress that the original working party was asked to produce criteria first without, at that stage, considering how they would be assessed. Most of the national criteria are to do with things that can be measured easily, such as the number of summaries in the medical records and audit activity. It is common knowledge that concentrating only on measurable items means that crucial aspects of a general practitioner's work are missed. This meant that the working party was not constrained in any way and the members' imaginations were subsequently challenged to devise new ways of assessing activities in the practice.

Evaluation

When the new arrangements were introduced it was agreed that after a pilot lasting 6 months they should be evaluated. Data were collected from the visiting team leaders, the doctors being assessed (before they knew the outcome of the visit) and each local trainers' group.[6] The main finding in relation to criteria was that they were acceptable but regular reviews would be necessary to ensure flexibility. The definition of the word 'standard' was raised and this has been referred to earlier.

The team

It has already been pointed out that, strictly speaking, the criteria and standards related to the trainer and not to the other people in the team. Nevertheless, it was possible to write statements that reflected good practice without treading on other professionals' toes. Relevant criteria read 'The teaching practice should be committed to teamwork. It should have close working relationships with district nurses, health visitors, midwives and social workers'.

Assessment methods

Once criteria and standards, or levels of performance, have been written and agreed, it is possible to decide how a practice will be assessed. In the case of Oxford in the 1980s the trainer working party was asked to plan a new method, which has largely stood the test of time since and has been used as the basis for trainer approvals in other places, including the Armed Forces GP training practices.[7]

It was clear at the outset that most of the relevant information came from a visit to the practice rather than from an interview with the trainer elsewhere. In this case it is possible to see examples of what is happening at first hand and to interview other people. Others can confirm what the trainer says, or not, as the case may be. In this case it is possible to see medical records and registers at first hand, to look at the library and audit projects. It was agreed therefore that, when the new arrangements were introduced in Oxford in the 1980s, visits should become routine and interviews dispensed with, except in rare circumstances. In fact, central interviewing in the region has now been given up altogether.

Equally important, a visit enables the visitors to talk with the other team members. From the outset, visitors asked to see health visitors, district nurses, midwives and practice managers, and it has been rare for anyone to refuse, except for unavoidable reasons. It is possible after a morning set of meetings to know how well the team works together and to what extent the non-medical members contribute to the teaching of the registrar. In general, these discussions have been appreciated by the people concerned and they have usually been keen to contribute to the compilation of the report.

During a visit it is also possible (and necessary) to interview the registrar, to find out how much teaching is being provided by the trainer, how well the practice provides a learning environment and what teaching is provided by people other than the doctors. In recent years there has been increasing emphasis on teaching by a variety of professionals. Primary healthcare is now given by teams whose members' boundaries are becoming increasingly blurred, and registrars need to see this and learn how it works. It is also good practice educationally for the registrar to learn from a variety of sources. Also, the use of a variety of professionals in teaching is a good model of teamwork for the registrar to observe.

The central part of any general practitioner's work is the consultation. It is therefore important to see consultations at first hand, partly because an assessment of the consultation can be made and partly because it is essential to know how the trainer uses consultations for teaching. Nevertheless, in the early 1980s it was with some trepidation that a decision was taken by the working party to introduce video-recorded consultations as part of the assessment procedure. The fact that it was accepted was due in no small part to the original work being done at the time, which has been referred to earlier.[3] This development had included clear guidelines for feeding back to the doctor the visitors' views in a constructive and positive way. In this, the visitors modelled what they expected to see from the trainer. The use of videotape was made easier by the development of new, small video cameras, which could be sited relatively unobtrusively in the doctor's consulting room. Nevertheless, some regions were still not using video recordings for trainer assessments a decade later.

Most regions use a standard report form, which should reflect the criteria and standards. It also ensures some standardisation between one set of visitors and another and reduces the likelihood that parts will be forgotten. It should also ensure that one report can be compared with the previous one.

In most regions the assessors are chosen from a small bank of experienced general practitioners. In some cases these are associate advisers in general practice, in others representatives of the local medical committee or a combination of the two. This should ensure that with a small number of people carrying out all the visits there is comparability between one visit and another. In Oxford a different method was adopted. Because people learn as much from visiting another practice as they do from being visited themselves, it was decided after the pilot scheme to ask all trainers to be part of visiting teams in another part of the region. This also introduced a peer review system so that doctors were being assessed by their colleagues rather than by a small group who might be seen as unrepresentative of general practice as a whole.

It also means that trainers learn the skills of making judgements about a practice and how to give feedback in a way that is both supportive and challenging. In the decade and a half that these arrangements have been working it has been highly successful, and the opportunities that it has created have been generally welcomed.

It was necessary, however, to ensure that a certain level of professionalism and skill was adopted. Trainers were allocated to teams, each one under an experienced leader, who was either the director, his deputy or associates, or a senior GP vocational trainer course organiser. In the very rare situation of a trainer potentially losing approval, a specially constructed team was sent to carry out the assessment.

In the early 1990s it was suggested at an annual trainers' meeting that it might be productive to introduce other team members to the visits. This suggestion was taken up and a pilot scheme of practice managers joining the visiting team was set up. The managers are treated as full members of the team, although they do not sit in on the trainer's interview or the viewing of the video-recorded consultations. The usual plan is for the practice manager to deal with the administrative aspects of the practice, including interviewing most of the administrative staff. She or he normally sits in on the interview with the partners and the registrar. Over lunch it is possible for the visitors to pool their findings. This has meant that findings can be confirmed or, alternatively, where there is disagreement or lack of information the manager can be asked to investigate further while the doctors are conducting the trainer interview. One of the advantages of these arrangements is that the practice managers see a different aspect of the practice and people will often say things to a manager that they will not say to doctors. This enables the team to build up a more comprehensive picture of what is going on and to cross-check information. The managers are also far better than the doctors at picking up matters to do with such things as health and safety and employment requirements.

An evaluation into the use of practice managers on practice visits was carried out, using questionnaires administered to the visiting assessors and the practice team being visited.[8] Over 90% of the latter felt comfortable with having a practice manager in the assessors and over 77% felt it was helpful. The only area where about half the practices were unhappy with the use of a manger was the inspection of individual patient records, although the majority had no problem with the managers looking at aggregated computerised data.

Ninety-nine per cent of the assessing doctors felt that their teams with a manager had been cohesive. The managers felt that there were three areas where they could contribute to the report which were not fully appreciated by the team leaders. These were the attitudes of the partners to training, the working environment and other aspects of the practice.

A selection and training programme was established by the practice managers themselves with support from the Director of Postgraduate GP Education. Each new manager was required to go on one or two visits with another manager before taking part in a visit on her or his own. Training and development days were held once or twice a year, when all team leaders and practice managers met to discuss current aspects of their work together with future changes.

The visit programme

It has been argued that for trainers to get the most value from the visit they need feedback on what is going well and what needs to be done, in a constructive way. It has also been argued that, in order to acquire an accurate picture, the visitors need to be in the building long enough to get all the information they need. They need to see members of the team and they need to cross-check data from one area with that from another.

The programme for a day's visit, which includes a practice manager in the visiting team, might look something like this:

08.30	Arrive. Team assemble. Tour premises.
09.00	Doctors interview attached staff while the practice manager interviews his or her counterpart.
09.30	Two doctors and the practice manager interview the registrar.
10.00	Doctors interview practice nurses while the practice manager interviews receptionists.
10.30	Coffee.
11.00	Team interviews partners.
11.45	Doctors inspect records, registers and library. Practice manager inspects computer system and checks other data.
12.30	Team confers over sandwich lunch in private.
13.30	Doctors interview trainer and view videotaped consultations or a videotaped tutorial. Practice manager checks on queries that have arisen from the morning and has a further session with his or her counterpart.
15.00	Team confers again and agrees main celebration areas and recommendations.
15.20	Doctors feed back to trainer.
15.30	Team feeds back to practice.
15.45	Leave.

A report is subsequently sent to the trainer and practice for checking for factual accuracy.

Evaluation

After pilot visits along these lines were introduced in the 1980s, there was general welcome for the process in the evaluation carried out in Oxford.[6] However, the logistical problem of visits lasting a whole day was identified and, partly as a result but more importantly because of the peer review process referred to earlier, the use of all trainers in the region was introduced. All except six readily agreed.

Trainers found being a member of a visiting team a valuable experience. Some staff found the visit stressful and the need for proper briefing was stressed. Health visitors, district nurses and practice nurses welcomed the opportunity to meet the visitors. The new arrangements meant that an adequate number of records could be examined instead of only a handful, which had often happened previously.

When the arrangements were introduced one trainer was not happy about the use of a video camera in his consulting room, but agreed to let one of the visitors sit in with him. Since then, no trainer has refused. Strict guidelines have been introduced by the General Medical Council to ensure that patients' informed consent is obtained for any video-recorded consultations. Videotaping is in regular use in all training practices now because of the requirement that all registrars submit taped consultations for certification purposes.

Impact and follow-up

Apart from the original papers published from Oxford in the 1980s[4,6,7], the number of publications on approval of trainers and training practices has been relatively sparse. Each region has looked at its criteria and methods periodically, with or without widespread consultation with its trainers. By the mid-1990s, there were still regions where the approval visits were carried out by a small group of general practitioners, usually associate advisers in general practice. Visits in some regions were still lasting only an hour or two. Some of this has reflected the contrasting views of those who believe the process is simply for a pass or fail decision and those who believe that the most important feature for the trainer and his or her colleagues is a detailed analysis of their strengths and areas for development.

For most practices, a training practice approval visit is the only detailed assessment by their peers that they get in the course of their daily work. A detailed report seems to have been appreciated by those involved. The introduction of practice managers to the visiting team, at least in one region, has gone some way to enhancing the team aspects of the visit and improving the quality and range of the feedback.

Costs

Perhaps the most frequent criticism of the visiting method established in Oxford was that it was too costly in terms of manpower, with three general practitioners being out of their practices for a whole day. Some of these doctors had to travel a fair distance since none of them visited practices within their own training-scheme area. In addition, the team leader had to compile a detailed report for the practice and the appointments committee.

Because all the trainers in the region were involved, on average each of them was involved in a visit once a year, and a few would do two. As part of their ongoing development, a visit to a colleague's practice can legitimately be seen as an integral part of the job for which a grant is being paid. Equally, for the director and adviser team, who comprise a substantial part of the team leaders, one visit four times a year is not only educational but enables them to stay in touch with training practice development. A small group of trainers and course organisers, who make up the remainder of the team leaders, are paid a daily rate, since this work is not part of their job description and involves more than simply doing the visit. All practice managers are paid a daily rate.

National guidelines require that no new practice can be approved for more than 2 years and no re-approval can last for more than 5 years. Many regions reduce the latter period, and in Oxford's case it is currently 4 years. A significant number of practices are re-approved but not for the full amount of time possible. With around 100 training practices in the Oxford region, on average between 36 and 40 visits are carried out each year.

The other consideration is what a region considers is a reasonable amount of time to allocate to this exercise in relation to all the other activities it has to undertake. The view in Oxford is that, considering the influence a training practice has on the individual registrars attached to it (bearing in mind that this is the only postgraduate training attachment most of the registrars will have), a full day reviewing its performance every 2–4 years is not excessive. With widely scattered training practices, it has to be remembered that, if conducted well, approval visits are one of the ways in which a region maintains some cohesiveness amongst its teachers.

Conclusions

Training practice accreditation has been one of the success stories of British general practice. No other branch of the profession has developed such a detailed review system for its teachers that probes not only the service aspects of the practice but also the teaching ability of the trainer.

Several general points can be made as a result of two decades of development. First, criteria and standards must remain flexible and capable of reflecting changing patterns of primary healthcare. Secondly, any process of judgement about a practice must have an effective, built-in feedback mechanism, so that the whole team can receive praise and recommendations. Thirdly, the process must reflect the fact that primary healthcare is increasingly delivered by a team and not by individuals. Fourthly, any system must involve the people being assessed, and not simply be imposed, if it is to be successful.

At a time when health professionals are feeling increasingly stressed from external pressure to deliver high-quality care, the development of training practice assessment has been one of the landmark developments from which we have learned much. General practice can be justifiably proud of what it has achieved.

1 Hasler JC (1982) Shortlisting trainees – overwhelmed in Oxford. *BMJ*. **285**: 1705–6.

2 Joint Committee on Postgraduate Training for General Practice (1980) *Criteria for the Selection of Trainers in General Practice*. JCPTGP, London.

3 Pendleton D, Schofield T, Tate P and Havelock P (1984) *The Consultation – An Approach to Learning and Teaching*. GP Series 6. Oxford University Press, Oxford.

4 Schofield TPC and Hasler JC (1984) Approval of trainers and training practices in the Oxford region: criteria. *BMJ*. **288**: 538–40.

5 Royal College of General Practitioners (1985) *What Sort of Doctor?* Report from General Practice 23. RCGP, London.

6 Schofield TPC and Hasler JC (1984) Approval of trainers and training practices in the Oxford region: evaluation. *BMJ*. **288**: 688–99.

7 Schofield TPC and Hasler JC (1984) Approval of trainers and training practices in the Oxford region: assessment. *BMJ*. **288**: 612–14.

8 Johnson N, Hasler J, Hobden-Clarke L and Bryceland C (1997) The role of a practice manager on training practice assessment visits. *Education for General Practice*. **8**: 128–34.

7

An evaluation of the RCGP team-based practice accreditation programme

Nicola Walsh and Kieran Walshe

In 1997, the Health Services Management Centre at the University of Birmingham was commissioned to conduct an evaluation of the pilot programme of team-based practice accreditation being established by the Royal College of General Practitioners (which was described in some detail in Chapter 4). This chapter presents some of the key findings from the study, which has been reported in detail elsewhere.[1] Evaluations of accreditation programmes are by no means commonplace, and so this study provides a useful insight into the workings of accreditation programmes and their place in primary care, which is probably of wider relevance.

Study design

The overall aim of the study was to assess the validity of the RCGP standards and criteria, the acceptability of the method of assessment, and the effectiveness of practice-based assessment in promoting changes in practice. There were two components to the study: an internal and an external perspective. The external component of the project was designed to assess the validity of the criteria and the accreditation process from the viewpoint of those working in and with primary care services in England. The internal component aimed to examine the validity, reliability and utility of the criteria and the accreditation process from the viewpoint of those involved in the pilot programme. The two strands of the evaluation took place in parallel.

Several data collection methods were used in the study. In the external component part of the study, focus groups were conducted to elicit the views of those working in or with primary care towards the standards and assessment process of the RCGP scheme. The focus groups were held in six health authorities across England. The six authorities were selected randomly from a stratified sampling frame to reflect the different levels of expertise in accreditation across the health authorities. Some authorities had no experience of accreditation, others had some experience of accreditation but not in primary care, and some had done a lot of work in primary care accreditation. A questionnaire seeking people's views on the RCGP criteria was also distributed to focus-group members.

In the internal component of the study, data were collected through semi-structured interviews with key personnel in the participating practices, before the visit, shortly after the visit and 6 months later. Data were also collected through non-participant observation of some of the accreditation visits, a review of the completed accreditation documentation, and from an analysis of the practices' self-assessment against the standards, individual assessor's ratings and the combined assessor's ratings.

Evaluation findings

The key findings from this evaluation study are presented in relation to:

- the validity, reliability and measurability of the standards and criteria

- the reliability of the assessment
- the acceptability of the method of assessment
- the effectiveness of practice-based assessment in promoting changes in the practice.

The full results of the evaluation study are available.[1]

The validity, reliability and measurability of the standards and criteria

The validity of the standards and criteria

The validity of the standards is central to the value of any accreditation programme. In the focus-group discussions, it was generally felt that there was little research evidence to support many of the standards and criteria. This did not mean that focus-group members necessarily disagreed with the standards and criteria concerned, and indeed some were held to be so self-evident as to probably not require, or be capable of, further proof. However, it was argued that the more contentious standards could easily be challenged because they represented, at best, a professional consensus about good practice and were not supported by rigorously conducted research. The standards concerned with appointment systems and appointment times were cited frequently as examples.

Some criteria were criticised for being not particularly relevant or appropriate to some practices, or in some settings. It was felt that where criteria defined, or were based around, particular processes, there could often be other ways of doing things that achieved the same outcome but in different ways. The standards and criteria did not necessarily allow for the justifiable diversity in practice that would be found in primary care, and this could result in practices being assessed as not meeting the criteria when they were actually providing good-quality care – a kind of technical rather than an actual breach of the standards.

The reliability of the standards and criteria

The reliability of some criteria – particularly where they used subjective adjectives or modifiers (such as 'appropriate', 'when relevant', 'if needed', 'as required', etc.) – was criticised by focus-group members. It was generally recognised that designing wholly objective and measurable criteria was difficult, and had some drawbacks itself, in that such criteria might be very rigid, and oriented towards measuring the most obviously measurable things. Criteria sometimes needed to embody ideas or principles that were important, but difficult to measure. The standard concerned with team values was often cited as an example.

It was widely believed that if the intention of the accreditation programme was measurement for accountability's sake, then the reliability of criteria was all-important, and imprecise, ambiguous or unquantifiable standards and criteria needed to be removed or modified. If, on the other hand, the purpose was primarily developmental, then it was important that themes such as team values were retained, and the measurability of the criteria mattered less than the ideas they embodied.

Focus-group members were asked to complete a detailed questionnaire about the standards and criteria, aimed at finding out how valid they felt they were. For each criterion, focus-group members were asked to indicate whether or not they felt it should be used in accrediting practices. If they believed that it should, they were then asked to indicate what level of practice it represented, using a three-point scale – essential, good practice or desirable practice. In total, 50 (out of 72) participants in the focus-groups completed and returned a questionnaire.

Table 7.1 provides an overview of the results from this survey with focus-group members.

Table 7.1: Summary of ratings of standards in the questionnaire completed by focus-group members

Number	Standard	Whether criteria rated as 'should be used in assessment' (%)		
		Yes	No answer	No
1	Accessibility	92	2	6
2	Communication	86	3	11
3	Prescribing	86	4	10
4	Investigations	90	3	7
5	Preventive health services and health promotion	87	3	10
6	Chronic disease care	86	6	8
7	Children's health	86	5	9
8	Mental health services	77	5	18
9	Family planning and women's health	86	6	8
10	Maternity services	77	8	15
11	Continued care at home	83	7	10
12	Elderly surveillance	68	12	20
13	Minor operations	93	2	5
14	Team values	76	4	19
15	Training and continued learning	91	5	4
16	Teamworking	85	4	11
17	Records	90	4	6
18	Management	88	5	7
19	Quality assurance and audit	81	8	11
20	Premises	88	7	6
	All standards	86	5	9

In general, these results show quite good support for most of the standards from focus-group members. Across all standards, 86% of criteria were rated as 'should be used' (with 9% being rated as not suitable for use, and 5% not being rated by the respondent). In order to explore which criteria were least well accepted by members of the focus-groups, the ratings for all those criteria accepted by less than 75% of focus-group members were identified (Table 7.2).

Table 7.2: Ratings of criteria in the questionnaire to focus-group members that were accepted by less than 75% of respondents

Number	Criterion	Whether criterion rated as 'should be used in assessment' (%)		
		Yes	*No answer*	*No*
2.1	Average length of booked appointments is not less than 10 minutes	64	2	34
5.5	Team produces a profile of health needs and strategy for health inequalities	68	2	30
7.4	Parents hold record of children's health and team members offer to complete it	68	4	28
7.7	Team enhances parents' ability and confidence to care for children when ill	74	4	22
8.1	Team has strategies for detecting depression and alcohol problems	64	6	30
8.2	Patients with anxiety, depression and alcohol problems get treatment and non-pharmacological support	72	6	22
9.3	Women are offered choice of female doctor or nurse to take cervical smear	74	6	20
10.1	Team has policy for providing preconceptual advice	68	8	24
10.6	Women are encouraged to breast feed	74	8	18
10.7	The breast feeding rate is audited	58	8	34
11.2	Team works with social services and others to co-ordinate care	74	8	18

continued

12.1	Patients aged 75 or over are offered annual consultation or home visit for assessment	68	10	22
12.2	Assessment includes sensory functions, mobility, mental condition, physical condition and environment	66	14	20
12.3	Conclusions from assessments discussed with patients and carers	72	12	16
12.4	Needs identified guide planning and provision of team	66	12	22
14.1	Team is committed to working with individuals, groups and the community	72	6	22
14.4	Team develops in response to new needs, has critical self-scrutiny, maintains skills	72	4	24
14.5	Team members maintain their physical and mental health and keep in bounds their need to be needed	52	6	42
16.9	Team members have identified sources of support both within and outside the team	66	4	30

It can be seen that no criterion was actually rejected by focus-group members but some had quite low acceptance ratings. Those given low ratings reflected concerns about the validity of some criteria (such as 2.1 and 5.5, on length of appointments and health needs assessment) and the reliability or measurability of others (such as 14.5, on team members' personal health).

The measurability of the standards and criteria

At each practice, the assessors rated the practice against the standards and criteria, first as individuals and then combining their ratings into a consensus view among their team. Prior to the assessment visit, each practice had rated itself against the standards and criteria. An analysis of these ratings is presented in Table 7.3 and is used to examine the validity and reliability of the standards and criteria.

Table 7.3: Assessors' ratings of compliance with the standards by the pilot practices

Number	Standard	Whether criteria rated as 'should be used in assessment' (%)		
		Yes	No answer	No
1	Accessibility	97	1	2
2	Communication	93	5	2
3	Prescribing	75	8	17
4	Investigations	98	0	2
5	Preventive health services and health promotion	92	0	8
6	Chronic disease care	88	0	11
7	Children's health	99	0	1
8	Mental health services	85	4	10
9	Family planning and women's health	88	1	11
10	Maternity services	87	1	12
11	Continued care at home	95	0	5
12	Elderly surveillance	98	0	2
13	Minor operations	70	8	22
14	Team values	100	0	0
15	Training and continued learning	97	3	0
16	Teamworking	87	2	11
17	Records	93	1	6
18	Management	84	4	12
19	Quality assurance and audit	75	2	23
20	Premises	88	2	10
	All standards	91	2	7

It can be seen that while overall compliance was high (91% of criteria were met across all practices), it varied considerably from standard to standard. Compliance was lowest for the standards on prescribing, minor operations and quality assurance and audit (3, 13 and 19). It is interesting to note the apparently complete compliance with standard 14 (team values), which contains some quite challenging but difficult-to-measure criteria. It may be that assessors were reluctant to suggest a practice did not comply with these criteria because they were too difficult measure.

The proportion of 'no answer' ratings varied from standard to standard, and it seemed that assessors had used this to indicate uncertainty – either about whether the standard was met or whether it was appropriate to the practice concerned. The highest levels of 'no answer' ratings were found for two of the standards in which compliance was in any case poor – prescribing and minor operations (3 and 13).

The level of compliance shown in Table 7.3 for each standard represents aggregate performance across the criteria contained within the standards, and there were some criteria with which compliance was particularly low. Criteria not met by the majority of practices concerned the auditing of minor operations and the use of staff appraisal.

Assessment against the standards did produce a range of performance, and so in that sense the RCGP accreditation programme did provide a discriminating measure or instrument, capable of differentiating one practice from another. Whether that differentiation is valid, measuring real and meaningful differences between practices, is very difficult to tell, without some other measure with which to compare it.

The reliability of assessment

The reliability of the assessments was explored in two ways: by comparing the assessor teams' rating with practices' own self-assessments, and by comparing the ratings made by individual assessors of a practice before they agreed on a joint rating.

Each practice assessed its own performance against the standards, in advance of its accreditation visit. The practice self-assessment was made available to the team of assessors before their visit, so they were aware of the practice self-assessment ratings when they undertook their own ratings. Each team of three assessors was asked during the visit firstly to rate the practice against the criteria and standards individually at first, without comparing notes, and then to agree together a consensus rating of the practice.

Table 7.4 presents a comparison of the rates of compliance with the criteria within each standard by practices reported by the assessor teams and reported by practices' self-assessments. It is immediately obvious that practices tended to assess themselves more favourably than the assessor teams – the mean rate of compliance was 96% according to practices themselves, compared with 91% according to the assessor teams. For the standards where assessor teams found the lowest levels of compliance (prescribing, minor operations and quality assurance and audit) there are substantial discrepancies. For example, assessor teams found a 75% rate of compliance with the criteria within the prescribing standard, while practices had reported 100% compliance (in other words, that they met all the criteria).

It appears that assessors quite often formed a different view about practices' compliance with the standards from that which the practices themselves held before the accreditation visit (or, at least, which they reported). In this light, it might have been expected that many practices would challenge the assessors findings, but they did not. It seems more likely that practices were rather generous to themselves in their own assessments, interpreting criteria in ways that allowed them to conclude that they met the criteria or standards concerned.

The presence of such a systematic bias (practice self-assessment ratings being consistently higher than assessors' ratings) inevitably affects the apparent reliability of the criteria and standards. We examined reliability by comparing the assessments made for each criterion and for each practice by the assessors and by the practice themselves.

Table 7.4: Comparison of compliance with standards as measured by assessor's ratings and practice self-assessment

Number	Standard	Compliance with criteria within standard (%)	
		Assessor Ratings	*Practice self-assessment*
1	Accessibility	97	98
2	Communication	93	97
3	Prescribing	75	100
4	Investigations	98	100
5	Preventive health services and health promotion	92	96
6	Chronic disease care	88	100
7	Children's health	99	99
8	Mental health services	85	91
9	Family planning and women's health	88	94
10	Maternity services	87	88
11	Continued care at home	95	96
12	Elderly surveillance	98	100
13	Minor operations	70	85
14	Team values	100	99
15	Training and continued learning	97	91
16	Teamworking	87	97
17	Records	93	95
18	Management	84	94
19	Quality assurance and audit	75	98
20	Premises	88	98
	All standards	91	96

It will be remembered that each criterion was rated on whether it was met, with answers of 'Yes', 'No' or 'No answer' being recorded. Because both assessors and practices had used the 'No' and 'No answer' options inconsistently, sometimes recording no answer to indicate uncertainty of decision as well as lack of knowledge, we grouped these two options together and then calculated how frequently practices and assessors had agreed or disagreed about their rating. These raw agreement percentages for the criteria within each standard are listed in Table 7.5

Because some level of agreement will always happen by chance, the raw agreement statistics are not a particularly good guide to the reliability of measurement. The kappa statistic, κ, is a measure of how far agreement exceeds that which would be expected by chance, and is a more useful indicator of the reliability of measurement.[2] If $\kappa = 0$, then the level of agreement is no more than that which would be expected by chance, while $\kappa = 1$ indicates perfect reliability. Negative values of κ represent less agreement than would be expected even through chance, and can be difficult to interpret. A commonly used rule of thumb is that values of κ of 0.81 or more represent very good reliability; the range 0.61–0.80 indicates good reliability, values between 0.41 and 0.60 represent moderate reliability, values from 0.21 to 0.40 show fair reliability and values of κ of 0.20 or less indicate poor reliability.[3] The values of κ for each standard are also listed in Table 7.5. Note that in some cases κ could not be calculated, because of the highly skewed distribution of the data (with many 'Yes' values, and few or even no 'No/no answer' values).

It can be seen that the overall value of κ for all standards is 0.26, which represents fair reliability. Only 5 of the 20 standards have κ values in the range 0.41 to 0.6, indicating moderate reliability, and none would be rated as showing either good or excellent reliability. Of course, these indications of relatively low reliability were in part to be expected, given that some systematic bias in the use of the accreditation standards by practices and assessors was found, with practices rating their compliance higher than assessors.

It was noted earlier that the three members of each assessor team made their own individual assessments of practices' compliance with the criteria and standards, before working together to agree the consensus rating used in the above analysis. The analysis of reliability for a pair of individual ratings for each practice was repeated and the statistical values for each standard are presented in Table 7.6.

Table 7.5: Comparison of assessor ratings and practice self-assessment by standard, showing raw percentage agreement and statistical measure of agreement

Number	Standard	Agreement between assessor and practice ratings	
		Raw agreement (%)	Kappa statistic κ
1	Accessibility	98	0.56
2	Communication	95	0.47
3	Prescribing	76	–
4	Investigations	98	–
5	Preventive health services and health promotion	95	0.55
6	Chronic disease care	87	–
7	Children's health	98	-0.01
8	Mental health services	84	0.28
9	Family planning and women's health	90	0.43
10	Maternity services	87	0.43
11	Continued care at home	91	-0.05
12	Elderly surveillance	98	–
13	Minor operations	76	0.37
14	Team values	98	–
15	Training and continued learning	88	-0.05
16	Teamworking	85	0.07
17	Records	91	0.25
18	Management	83	0.22
19	Quality assurance and audit	75	0.11
20	Premises	89	0.22
	All standards	90	0.26

Table 7.6: Comparison of individual assessor ratings by standard, showing raw percentage agreement and statistical measure of agreement

Number	Standard	Agreement between individual assessor ratings	
		Raw agreement (%)	Kappa statistic κ
1	Accessibility	87	0.03
2	Communication	89	0.44
3	Prescribing	77	0.49
4	Investigations	77	0.17
5	Preventive health services and health promotion	88	0.45
6	Chronic disease care	76	0.38
7	Children's health	67	-0.06
8	Mental health services	55	-0.03
9	Family planning and women's health	63	0.11
10	Maternity services	73	0.41
11	Continued care at home	68	0.21
12	Elderly surveillance	77	0.17
13	Minor operations	70	0.40
14	Team values	92	-0.04
15	Training and continued learning	91	-0.10
16	Teamworking	86	0.49
17	Records	60	0.02
18	Management	64	0.27
19	Quality assurance and audit	70	0.25
20	Premises	92	0.73
	All standards	75	0.27

The overall κ statistic of 0.27 again represents fair reliability. In this case, 6 of the 20 standards have κ values of 0.41 – 0.60 (representing moderate reliability) and just one has a κ value between 0.61 and 0.80 (representing good reliability).

These analyses suggest that the criteria and standards as they stand are difficult to apply and use reliably, and that different assessors are likely to produce significantly different ratings for the same practice. The low reliability suggests that these measures should not be used as a basis for significant decisions or actions (such as a decision to give or deny accreditation status) without further corroboration or supporting evidence from other sources.

The acceptability of the method of assessment

The method of assessment used in the RCGP team-based accreditation programme has been described in detail in Chapter 4. To summarise, there are three phases: the pre-assessment preparation phase, the assessment visit and the feedback.

The pre-assessment phase

Without doubt, the prospect of the accreditation visit in many of the participating practices, and the preparations required, created a feeling of enthusiasm and excitement, which the GPs and the practice managers were able to use to enhance teamwork.

A major benefit arising from the requirement to provide information before the visit was that practice staff were able to review and amend information systems and processes. A perhaps unintended benefit of the preparation process was that it required the collation of policies and statistical information that, in many cases, had not been collected before in one central point. Many of the practices reported that the process of preparation had created greater awareness amongst all staff about current procedures,

'I've learnt a lot I'm much more aware of what goes on in the practice...'

'The process of going through the standards has been used to create greater awareness amongst practice staff about current procedures.'

This pre-assessment phase appears to have given staff legitimate 'time out' from their busy workload to look at the organisation of the practices as a whole and not just their own contribution.

The accreditation visit

The purpose of the one-day visit is to verify the information that has been sent to the assessors in the pre-assessment documentation and to survey the practice. The visit is conducted by a team of three, a GP, a practice nurse and a practice manager. They collect a range of data at the visit to enable them to see how the practice operates. To do this, they used a range of surveying techniques: non-participant observation, interviewing and documentation review. At the visit, time was short so the assessors worked separately, looking at different parts of the practice. This mode of working proved to be economical in time and was far less obtrusive for patients and staff. One assessor usually sat with the reception staff, while another spent some time with the practice manager, and the third assessor (normally the general practitioner) began to interview some of the practice staff.

The overall aim of the interviews was to gain an insight into staff attitudes and to gather a bit more information about how they worked in the practice. In the assessors guidance it was suggested that the interview should take the form of an informal chat rather than a structured interview. As skilled interviewers know, this is no easy task. A non-structured interview requires an enormous amount of preparation beforehand. The interviewers need to be familiar with their material, in this case the pre-assessment information that had been sent a few weeks before the visit.

While the assessors in the Brent and Harrow pilot programme were given some guidance about the questions they should ask, some did admit to us that they did find it rather difficult to adopt a conversational rather than an interrogative style of interviewing. Some of the practice staff did complain to us about the style and content of the interviews,

'The interviews did not address the specifics and so some of the key issues were missed. An assessor needs a definite plan.'

'Some of the staff found the assessors interviewing skills threatening.'

'One of the nurses felt threatened by the questions of the nurse assessor.'

Interview training for assessors is a key issue that needs to addressed more in any future programme.

Patient records were also assessed for completeness, accuracy, legibility, order, childhood immunisation and elderly surveillance rates, other documentation, such as the minutes of practice meetings, audit results, protocol and practice policies, was also reviewed by assessors. The practice's self-assessment forms gave assessors an indication of how the practice perceived itself against the criteria, and the practice questionnaire gave them some background information about the practice. The questionnaire also provided assessors with information about how the practice fared against the criteria, as many of the criteria had been turned into questions. The data collected from all these different information sources were collated at the end of the day and used by the assessors to consider whether or not the practice had complied sufficiently with the standards.

One difficulty with any accreditation programme is that much of the evaluation relies on the value judgements of the assessors. Do the assessors think it is a good practice or not? Were they impressed by the general ambience of the practice? Did they get the right answers to the questions they asked? Did they in fact ask the right questions? On the whole, the practices felt that the assessors were very thorough, acted professionally and were very supportive. All the practices reported that surgeries ran as normal, and that there were no complaints from the patients.

'The assessors turned up on time, they were efficient and polite.'

'The visit went well the assessors turned up on time...no one felt threatened.'

'The surgeries ran as normal, we hardly noticed they were there.'

'The visit went well, the assessors stuck to the fairly tight timetable.'

The main concerns were that in some instances the assessors missed pieces of information and were therefore given the impression that some of the things were not being done when they were.

Some practices found the accreditation visit a nerve-racking experience, although they enjoyed it. Many said they felt tired at the end of the day and experienced a feeling of anticlimax. One practice celebrated 'getting through' the day by opening a bottle of champagne. Some of the staff were upset by the visit and felt that the comments made by the assessors had been unfair.

Feedback

At the end of the visit, the team of assessors discussed their findings amongst themselves and then presented these back to the practice staff. This verbal feedback was to provide an opportunity for staff to comment on the assessment and to challenge any findings they considered to be inaccurate. In the guidance, the assessors had been asked to begin their feedback with a general overview of the practice. They had also been asked to alternate between those services considered to be good and those which were seen to be a problem. There were mixed views about the value of the feedback at the end of the day. Some felt that it had been very useful and that the assessors had been constructive.

'The verbal feedback went well...I had not realised how much they would feed back.'

'The verbal feedback went fine. The comments and criticism were useful. Nothing was unexpected.'

Whereas, some interviewees felt that the feedback was not as thorough as it could have been,

> 'The verbal feedback at the end of the day was not constructive enough.'

> 'All the assessors contributed to the feedback – it was relatively bland and did not rock any boats.'

Some practice staff felt inhibited and did not feel they could disagree with the feedback,

> 'The verbal feedback was too directive and opinionated and I felt it was insensitively handled.'

> 'Personally, I felt inhibited I did not want to disagree with them.'

The style of the feedback varied enormously. In some cases the feedback was given by all three of the assessors, but more frequently one person led the feedback, with the other members contributing in their areas of expertise. Attendance at the feedback by practice staff did vary. In some there were no doctors present at all, whereas in others, the GPs were keen to protect their staff, so the feedback was just given to the partners and the practice manager. Some of these GPs fed back the results to staff at the next practice meeting, others did not.

The aim of the written report was to provide an account of the assessors' findings and illustrate the practice's performance against criteria. To facilitate the production of the report the assessors were provided with a pro forma. The team leader was responsible for writing the report in consultation with the other team members. The production of the report often took longer than the allowed 2 weeks to complete. Some interviewees complained that they had to wait too long to receive their report,

> 'I thought we would have the report in a couple of weeks but the fact that we are still waiting means that it has lost a bit of its weight.'

'The real weakness has been in the delay in getting the written report.'

Certainly, some of the practice staff felt very strongly that the time between the visit and the report being received should not be any longer than 2–3 weeks, otherwise the momentum in the practice would be lost. Generally, the reports were felt to be acceptable documents, although one or two practices felt that they were too short.

'The written report arrived quickly – it was short but covered all the main points. It accurately reflected the verbal feedback.'

'The report took two weeks plus to arrive – the practice manager would have liked more feedback and found the report too brief especially as we had taken some time to prepare.'

The distribution of the report amongst practice staff varied, often depending upon the result it conveyed. Practices were accredited if only all the essential criteria had been met. The Head of Quality and Professional Development from the health authority contacted any practice that did not comply with the standards, and where necessary, support was provided to enable the practice to comply with the standards set.

Overall, the method of assessment used by the RCGP team-based accreditation programme was felt to be acceptable by those involved in the pilot programme.

The effectiveness of the RCGP programme in promoting change in the practice

Measuring whether or not the RCGP accreditation programme promoted change in the practices was challenging. The diversity across the practices made assessing the impact of the scheme difficult. Even when the impacts could be measured, their attribution to accreditation rather than other factors was not always clear. The study took place amidst a series of policy announcements, such as the end of GP fundholding, the development of PCGs and the development of new arrangements for clinical governance in all healthcare providers (including primary care). Such announcements herald a period of rapid change within primary care, and such changes inevitably affected the practices taking part in this study.

Within each practice, a continuing process of change was also evident. Few practices were still the same at the end of the study (July 1998) – in terms of staff, structures, facilities and processes of care – as they were at the outset of the study in September 1997. For example:

- six of the 12 practices had seen changes in their partnership arrangements
- four practices reported significant changes in other practice staffing, such as the arrival of a new practice manager
- three practices had seen major changes in their premises – in one case, moving completely to newly equipped and established facilities, while two others had expanded their existing buildings
- three practices reported that they had either now secured status as a training practice or that they were in the process of applying to become a training practice.

The pace of change, both nationally and locally, inevitably made the task of evaluating the impact of the RCGP accreditation programme more difficult. Acknowledging these difficulties, we still felt it was important to assess the effectiveness of the RCGP programme in promoting change in the practices. We therefore analysed the written reports to identify the recommendations for change made by the assessors. We then asked interviewees at each practice about whether these recommendations had been accepted and acted upon when we undertook follow-up visits to practices about 6 months after their accreditation visit had taken place.

Practices were given between 5 and 19 recommendations in their written reports (on average, each practice had ten recommendations). Most, though not all, of the assessors' reports linked recommendations to particular criteria within the accreditation standards. A list of the more common issues raised and recommendations made is given in Table 7.7.

Table 7.7: Common issues and recommendations from assessors' reports

Criteria		Number	Typical recommendation
5.5	The team produces a profile of the health needs of their population and identifies their strategies for tackling inequalities in health	4	No profile developed; need to work on this
6.1	The team has developed protocols for the management of chronic diseases which are used to guide the care that they provide	4	Either no protocols developed or not being used; need to develop and use as appropriate
9.1	The rubella immune status of women of childbearing age is established and recorded and those who require immunisation are offered it	6	No systems for doing this, left to individual clinicians; need to put procedures in place
10.1	The team has an agreed policy for providing preconceptual advice	4	No policy or not being used; need to develop and/or use
10.7	The breast feeding rate is audited	5	No audit; need to undertake one and act on findings
13.3	The practice audits their minor operations against accepted guidelines	5	No audit; need to undertake one and act on findings
18.10	All team members are regularly appraised and personal learning plans are agreed	6	No system for appraisal in place or no records kept; need to institute system

| 18.13 | The practice adheres to statutory requirements, including the Health and Safety at Work Act and other regulations | 5 | Minor infringements of fire, storage or waste regulations; need to rectify |
| 20.5 | The practice has a library that is accessible to all team members and which contains up-to-date reference books, books relevant to primary care and recent copies of major medical and nursing journals | 6 | No library, or library stock out of date and not maintained, need to make library provision |

There were no particular criteria for which recommendations seemed to produce disagreements with the practice, but there were some common themes evident in the nature of the disagreement. First, practices disagreed because they felt that the assessors had misunderstood the situation in their practice and so misrepresented facts in the report. Secondly, practices disagreed because they felt that the recommendation from the assessors, and by implication the criteria, did not take account of the context of their practice. Thirdly, practices sometimes disagreed with the recommendations because they felt that the standard they were being asked to achieve was too difficult or demanding given the limited benefits that compliance would bring for them or their patients.

At our follow-up visit interviewees were asked to report what had been done to implement each of the recommendations contained in the assessor's report. We categorised their descriptions of actions and planned actions on a four-point scale:

1 No action had been taken yet to implement the recommendation.
2 Action had been planned to implement the recommendation, but had not yet taken place.

3 Action had been taken to implement the recommendation, but it was not yet complete.
4 Action had been taken to implement the recommendation, and it was now complete.

The results of this analysis are summarised in Figure 7.1. It can be seen that 23% of recommendations had been fully implemented by the time of our follow-up visit, while action was in progress though not complete for a further 27%. In other words, about half of all recommendations had produced some form of action by the practice within the 6 months following the visit. However, this varied substantially from practice to practice, with one practice having acted on all the recommendations with which it agreed (2 out of 2) while another had acted on just 17% (1 out of 6).

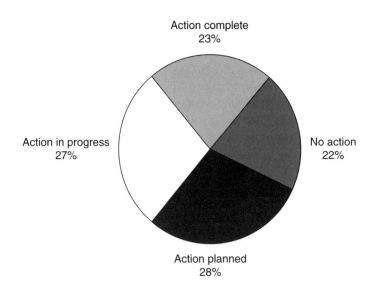

Figure 7.1 Implementation of actions recommended by assessors' reports with which practices agreed, across all practices.

While there were no particular criteria for which the recommendations had either been implemented or not, it was evident that the simpler and more administrative matters, such as the provision of equipment or the development of library provision had often been addressed, while some of the more intransigent or complex issues to do with clinical practice or team functioning were still outstanding.

Table 7.8 shows all the 21 recommendations for which action had been taken and completed – an average of less than two recommendations per practice. It can be seen that they are a heterogeneous group, some of which are relatively trivial in nature although others are more significant. However, it would probably be hard to justify the use of the accreditation process solely in terms of the impact implied in these changes.

Table 7.8: Recommendations for which action had been taken and completed by the time of the follow-up visits to practices

1   Non-attenders for breast screening clinic now being followed up.
2   Midwife now working in practice to provide antenatal care.
3   Main treatment room facilities upgraded.
4   Written records of practice meetings now being kept.
5   Various equipment for practice purchased.
6   Library stock of books and journals expanded.
7   Courses arranged to provide formal training for clerical staff.
8   Data protection registration/certificate for practice obtained.
9   Appraisal system developed, including assessment of training needs.
10 Storage of blood collection bottles changed to keep out of reach of children.
11 Now holding primary healthcare team meetings every 6 weeks and doctors meetings weekly.
12 Strategy for detecting depression now developed.
13 Minutes of practice meetings now being kept.
14 Library has been extended.
15 Warning signs about step down into nurses' room erected.
16 Thermometer placed in vaccine fridge.
17 Policies for preconceptual care and ascertaining rubella immune status of women developed and placed on computer.
18 Breast feeding rates audited.
19 Practice manager appointed.
20 Inadequate cervical smear rate audited.
21 Signposting of fire exits, etc. reviewed and improved.

It was clear from participants that, while change and improvement were important intended outcomes from their participation in this pilot programme of accreditation in primary care, these were far from being the sole or even primary purpose they had in mind, either at the outset, when they agreed to take part, or at the conclusion, when they looked back at the process in retrospect.

In broad terms, participants in this pilot programme supported the accreditation process, both beforehand and afterwards, and believed it to have been worthwhile for them and their practices. Of course, participants were, in part, a self-selected group likely to include those who enjoyed innovation and experimentation, and who supported the use of quality improvement mechanisms such as accreditation in primary care. So we should be cautious about concluding that other participants or potential participants in such a programme would share this generally positive assessment of the value of accreditation.

The pilot accreditation programme did indeed bring about some significant changes in the practices that took part, although it should be noted that only a minority of identified opportunities for change had been realised, and the nature of some of those changes was relatively small-scale and minor. Some of those changes, although we cannot tell what proportion, would have come about in any case, without the intervention of the accreditation programme.

The accreditation programme did produce a number of 'softer' benefits, such as the sharing of information across practices and between practice staff. The assessors also noted how valuable it had been to visit other practices. Overall, the 12 practices participating in the scheme remain positive about the value of accreditation and in general, found the programme beneficial.

Conclusions

The RCGP team-based practice accreditation programme has a number of important strengths, such as its focus on the practice (rather than on individual clinicians) as the unit for assessment, and its unique combination of using centrally developed standards with a locally managed accreditation process.

The evaluation study did, however, identify a number of ways in which the accreditation process could be improved. First, the standards and criteria could be revised, with a view to making their development and application more rigorous. Secondly, the assessment process could be improved by giving more training to assessors, focusing on how they are recruited and selected for the task, and more guidance on how to collect, analyse and feed back data from the assessments would be useful. Finally, more attention could be given to following up recommendations, either by practices themselves or by the accreditation programme.

1 Walsh N and Walshe K (1998) *Accreditation in Primary Care: an evaluation of the RCGP team-based practice accreditation programme.* University of Birmingham and RCGP, Birmingham.

2 Siegel S and Castellan J (1998) *Non-parametric Statistics for the Behavioural Sciences.* Second edition. McGraw-Hill, New York.

3 Brennan P and Silman A (1992) Statistical methods for assessing observer variability in clinical measures. *BMJ.* **304**: 1491–4.

8

Towards clinical governance: the future for accreditation

Theo Schofield, Kieran Walshe, Clare Blakeway-Phillips and Nicola Walsh

The approaches to accreditation in primary care described in the previous chapters of this book all predate the reforms to the NHS announced by the government in December 1997, including the development of primary care groups and a package of changes intended to improve the quality of health services.[1] These quality reforms, detailed in a consultation paper in July 1998,[2] set out a comprehensive portfolio of new structures, organisations and systems to set national standards for patient care, to deliver those standards at a local level through changes and improvements where necessary, and to monitor their implementation. This chapter explores where accreditation programmes fit into the new NHS, and especially how they might contribute to the development of clinical governance.

What is clinical governance?

Clinical governance is defined as 'a framework through which NHS organizations are accountable for continuously improving the quality of their services and safeguarding high standards of care by creating an environment in which excellence in clinical care will flourish'.[2] It is part of a new approach to quality in which those who lead NHS organisations will be held responsible for the quality of the services they provide, just as they have always been held responsible for their financial performance. To reinforce this point, a statutory duty for quality is to be established in law, the first time that such an explicit provision has been made in the legislation that governs the NHS.

The development of clinical governance seems to signal two key changes for NHS organisations. First, it is unambiguously clear that NHS organisations are corporately responsible for the quality of clinical care, and that accountability rests finally on their boards and chief officers. Secondly, NHS organisations are required to put in place systems for monitoring the quality of care, identifying and resolving or preventing problems, and stimulating improvements. It is no longer acceptable to provide health services without being able to ensure that a consistent and acceptable quality standard is met.

Clinical governance is perhaps the most important part of a framework of new systems and structures intended to make quality central to the agenda of the new NHS. Other elements include the following.

- National standards and guidance on the use of healthcare interventions from a new National Institute of Clinical Excellence (NICE), which may incorporate guidelines and standards set by other bodies, including the Royal Colleges, and will also direct a series of national audits of the quality of care.
- National service frameworks developed for particular major service areas or groups of patients, providing a template of service provision against which local healthcare providers can assess and review services. The first NSFs are on coronary heart disease and mental health.

- Continued support for professional self-regulation, with greater powers for the Secretary of State to review and strengthen existing and future professional registers. At the same time, professional bodies are generally moving towards new arrangements for dealing with poor clinical practice and procedures for the periodic renewal or reverification of clinicians' inclusion on professional registers. There will also be strong links between clinical governance and continuing professional development, with a requirement for NHS organisations to have development plans in place for all clinical staff.
- A new Commission for Health Improvement, tasked with inspecting local NHS trusts to ensure that adequate arrangements for clinical governance are in place and that national standards are being implemented appropriately.
- A national framework for assessing performance, consisting of new sets of performance indicators in six areas or dimensions, which will be used to compare or benchmark NHS trusts against each other and seek opportunities for improvement.

Taken together, this package of quality reforms can claim to be the most radical and far-reaching in the history of the NHS, capable of making quality of healthcare a central concern and high priority for clinicians, managers and patients.

The proposed structure for the delivery of clinical governance is that each trust or primary care group will have a designated senior clinician responsible for clinical governance, an executive member of the board with lead responsibility for clinical governance, and a board-level subcommittee responsible for clinical governance. They will also be expected to have a range of quality improvement programmes in place, including:

- full participation by all clinical professionals in audit programmes
- evidence-based practice, supported and applied routinely in everyday practice
- ensuring the clinical standards of National Service Frameworks and NICE recommendations are implemented

- workforce planning and development (i.e. recruitment and retention of appropriately trained workforce) fully integrated within their service planning
- continuing professional development programmes aimed at meeting the development needs of individual health professionals and the service needs of the organisation in place and supported locally
- appropriate safeguards to govern access to and storage of confidential patient information, as recommended in the Caldicott Report on the review of patient-identifiable information
- high-quality systems for clinical record keeping
- effective monitoring of clinical care in place and integrated with the quality programme for the organisation as a whole
- clear policies aimed at managing risks.

NHS trusts and PCGs will also be expected to have arrangements in place to identify and deal with any problems of poor performance, such as:

- critical incident reporting, ensuring that adverse events are identified and openly investigated, lessons are learned and promptly applied
- complaints procedures, accessible to patients and their families and fair to staff, in which lessons are learned and recurrence of similar problems avoided
- professional performance procedures, which take effect at an early stage before patients are harmed and which help the individual to improve his or her performance whenever possible, are in place and understood by all staff
- staff being supported in their duty to report any concerns about colleagues' professional conduct and performance, with clear statements from the Board on what is expected of all staff; there should be clear procedures for reporting concerns so that early action can be taken to support the individual and to remedy the situation.

The development of clinical governance has been paralleled by changes in the professional self-regulation machinery, particularly for doctors. The General Medical Council recently extended its powers to review poor clinical performance among doctors who, though not thought to be guilty of misconduct, are believed to fall below an acceptable standard of care in their practice and may present risks to patients. In 1999, the GMC took a further step towards tighter self-regulation, by agreeing in principle to introduce a process of periodic revalidation for all doctors. In short, medical practitioners will no longer be admitted to the Medical Register for life. In order to maintain their registration and license to practice, they will have to undergo a periodic review of their clinical performance and expertise. While the form of this process of revalidation has yet to be spelt out, it will undoubtedly draw on local arrangements for clinical governance, and locally collected data profiling the practice and proffessional development of each doctor.

Clinical governance in primary care

The proposals made for clinical governance in primary care are not as immediately demanding, nor as detailed, as those for NHS trusts. For example, trusts (but not PCGs) will be subject to visits from the Commission for Health Improvement once it is established, and must produce an annual published clinical governance report from March 2000 onwards.

This is quite understandable, since the fundamental changes in the structure of primary care heralded in the White Paper make it difficult to expect the same level of development in clinical governance in the short term. The introduction of primary care groups to which all practices will belong signals a very significant change in professional and managerial structures and cultures in primary care. Primary care groups will have wide responsibilities for budgeting, planning and for the delivery of clinical governance. It is envisaged that many primary care groups will develop into primary care trusts, by which time a full programme of clinical governance will need to be in place. Although, for the foreseeable future at least, general practices and their primary care teams will remain the unit of delivery of primary healthcare, the development of PCGs is likely to lead to a shift in the locus of clinical and managerial influence from individual practices to the new groups.

Primary care groups are new organisations, managed by a board made up of representatives of GPs, nurses, social services, health authorities and the public. There is a need for them to develop some sense of corporate identity and culture, even though the people within each PCG will continue to be employed by a number of different organisations.

Many of the activities proposed as part of clinical governance have been developed and are already being used in some places in primary care, including clinical audit, guidelines, risk-management-effective recording systems, critical incident monitoring and continuous quality improvement. However, it is undoubtedly true that none of these activities are universal, and perhaps the main challenge in the implementation of clinical governance in primary care is to spread existing good practice and see the development of the systems required in all practices, not just some or a few. It is important to remember the importance attached in current policy to tackling the unacceptable variations that exist in the quality of care received by patients, particularly in primary care.

The requirement from the General Medical Council to undergo periodic revalidation will apply to general practitioners, just as it does to hospital doctors. While NHS Trusts are likely to play a significant role in the process for the doctors they employ, it is much less clear to what extent primary care groups will be involved in revalidation for the general practitioners within the group. However, once again the local arrangements for clinical governance are likely to be an important source of data.

Accreditation and clinical governance

In this context, we now consider how the approaches to accreditation that have been described in earlier chapters of this book might contribute to the development of clinical governance. A number of key aims for clinical governance can be identified:

● fostering the organisational development of primary care teams and primary care groups

- improving the quality of patient care
- promoting individual professional development
- developing local ownership and involvement in quality improvement
- identifying and dealing with underperformance.

It was noted in Chapter 2 that for accreditation programmes to work effectively, it is very important that their aims are clearly defined and understood by all the stakeholders in the accreditation process. So it is important to consider how accreditation might contribute to each of the aims for clinical governance outlined above.

Does accreditation promote organisational development in primary care?

The development of primary care groups represents a shift from a partnership model of working, in which individual doctors, team members and practices retain a large degree of independence although they may well work together voluntarily, towards a more corporate model in which managers, whether they be doctors, nurses or professional managers, are responsible for the finance and the quality of the services that are provided, and are held accountable for them. If teamwork and partnership are replaced entirely by this corporate model, then many of the strengths of the present system of primary care will be lost, including the commitment of the professionals in the team to the development of their services to meet local needs. If, on the other hand, practices remain entirely independent, then unacceptable variations in the standard of care will persist. A balance between the two models is clearly needed.

Accreditation provides a way of linking traditional, professionally led systems of quality improvement with the new accountability that clinical governance demands. A system of professionally led assessment and quality development, based on an accreditation model with practices willing to accept external scrutiny from their colleagues, would, in our view, help to maintain the commitment of the primary care teams, and would also meet the needs of PCG boards to be assured of the quality of the services that they are providing. It would make an important contribution to building the organisational culture, structures and systems that PCGs need to fulfil their aims.

Does accreditation promote quality improvement in practice?

There is a growing recognition that there is no single mechanism for primary care teams to maintain and improve the quality of their services. There are many methods, including clinical audit, risk management, continuous quality improvement and so on, and no one approach is necessarily better or more effective than others. The key skill seems to be in selecting a method that suits the organisation and the problems to be addressed.

Accreditation can influence the quality of care directly by bringing about changes and improvements, as the evaluation reported in Chapter 7 demonstrated. However, it can also be used to assess the use and impact of other quality improvement mechanisms, through criteria focused in these areas. By combining a practice's own self-assessment of their progress in quality improvement with an external assessment, accreditation may help to promote quality improvement both directly and indirectly. The General Medical Council supports this in its publication on maintaining good medical practice,[3] which argues that practices should be 'testing themselves against others providing similar care, to see where they stand and to learn from this'.

Does accreditation encourage individual professional development?

It is accepted that individual healthcare professionals need to maintain their fitness to practice, which involves identifying their own learning needs and taking steps to meet them. Increasingly, however, this is seen as both a personal responsibility for the clinician and an organisational responsibility for the NHS organisation in which he or she works. The Chief Medical Officer's review of continued medical education recommended that clinicians' personal learning plans should be developed from practice development plans, so that continued professional development helps to maintain the quality of both the individual and the practice's performance. Accreditation, although focused on the organisation rather than the individual, provides an important opportunity to review and reassess practice development plans. Moreover, accreditation standards can contain criteria that directly assess the practice's systems for producing, updating and meeting personal learning plans.

Can accreditation promote local ownership of quality improvement?

The development of accreditation standards and criteria by national bodies has the advantage of avoiding duplication of effort, and the resulting criteria may command a reasonable degree of credibility as a result of the implied or actual endorsement by those organisations. A national set of standards may also help to promote equity in practice in different parts of the country. However, local circumstances do vary considerably and local involvement in standard setting and assessment are needed, both to enable the process to reflect the varying needs of practice teams and to make it more acceptable and feasible at a local level. The validity of these criteria is crucial to the credibility of this programme, and they will need to be continually updated in the light of new evidence and new developments.

Primary care groups that are multidisciplinary and include representatives of patients are well placed to set up local groups that can incorporate existing expertise in clinical audit and primary care development, and can implement a programme of practice accreditation. These assessments can form the basis of development plans for practices, individual team members and for the primary care group, and also enable the quality of services being provided to be assured. However, it would probably be unrealistic and undesirable for primary care groups to set about creating the standards and criteria for such an accreditation process for themselves, because of the investment of time and effort needed. PCGs need a set of standards and criteria that they can adapt and then adopt locally. These criteria can reflect both national priorities (such as NICE guidance and national service frameworks) and local activities required for quality improvement and risk management.

Primary care groups can provide the local co-ordination and support for a local accreditation programme, but may need support for assessor training and possibly a network of assessors external to the group to maintain the validity of the assessments. Attention would also need to be given to the rewards and incentives to individuals and teams to become involved in such a programme. There are positive gains from being assessed by one's colleagues and achieving high standards, and without clear targets motivation can diminish. However, professionals will always balance these gains against the costs, particularly the time involved, and the risks of criticism or failure. A supportive educational ethos is essential to minimise those risks. Overall, accreditation may be able to combine the best characteristics of national development (credibility, rigour and comparability) with local application (participation, ownership and support).

Does accreditation help to identify and deal with underperformance?

Accreditation may not be the best tool for dealing with known problems of poor performance, either in organisations or of individual clinicians. A more sensitive and individually tailored approach is more likely to be successful. However, accreditation can contribute to managing underperformance in two key ways. First, it can provide a diagnostic tool, capable of identifying performance problems at an early stage and signalling the need for action or intervention. Secondly, the regular use of some form of accreditation may prevent such problems developing, because it ensures that individuals and organisations are assessed by themselves and others against an objective and comparable benchmark and that plans for improvement are then put in place.

Accreditation and quality improvement

One issue that requires clarification is the relative merits of a system of accreditation in which the result is a pass or fail decision against a system in which the focus is on development and improvement, and participation rather than a particular standard of performance is the main measure used. Both have their advantages. For example, practices taking part in accreditation often want a formal 'pass' judgement to be made in order to validate their investment of time and effort in the process. On the other hand, pass/fail judgements can be difficult to reach, may deter or disadvantage poorer practices that are, nevertheless, trying hard to improve, and can end up dominating the accreditation process, of which they are only one small part.

The public, on the other hand, may demand a system that identifies underperforming professionals or teams, and there is considerable criticism of the track record of professional self-regulation. It is always difficult, but very important, to argue that the greatest good for the greatest number is achieved by involving all practices in making improvements in their care, rather than concentrating on identifying a small number of 'bad apples'. If the focus of accreditation is placed on quality improvement, it can involve the whole practice team in raising the quality of their patient care, can use criteria that are important, but not necessarily highly measurable, and can contribute to wider organisational and professional development.

Conclusions

Clinical governance requires NHS organisations to have robust and effective local systems for quality improvement, which enable them to meet national clinical standards. This requires a blend of national leadership and local ownership; and a combination of professional development and corporate accountability. We believe that an approach to clinical governance that made use largely of national standards and external inspection would not command the respect and support of many clinical professionals. However, leaving governance to local NHS organisations, without any national co-ordination and guidance, is likely to lead to duplication of effort and more rather than less, variation in practice. Moreover, one lesson of the evaluation reported in Chapter 7 is that when methods for quality improvement and clinical governance are developed, it is important that their impact and effectiveness are tested rigorously in practice. But this kind of evaluation is probably only feasible at a national or regional level.

A middle ground is needed, in which diversity and creativity are encouraged at a local level, and sufficient scope is allowed for local flexibility and differences in context, but in which there is also co-ordination and collaboration at a national level. Accreditation, especially where it is nationally sponsored but locally applied and managed, has much to offer in this regard. However, whatever approach to clinical governance PCGs choose to employ or develop, they need to take account of three fundamental principles that emerge from the experience of using accreditation in primary care. First, the quality of primary care depends most of all on the contributions of all members of the primary healthcare team and the way that they work together. Secondly, patients are entitled to be assured that these services are of high quality, and that systems are in place to ensure that quality is maintained and improved. Thirdly, the most effective ways of improving and assuring quality rely on a combination of professional education, development and regulation with organisational strategy, co-ordination and action. Clinical governance, if it is to succeed, has to bring together the best of the professional and managerial cultures.

1 Department of Health (1997) *The New NHS: Modern, Dependable*. The Stationery Office, London.

2 Department of Health (1998) *A First Class Service: quality in the new NHS*. Department of Health, London.

3 General Medical Council (1998) *Maintaining Good Medical Practice*. GMC, London.

Appendix

RCGP standards and criteria for accreditation

These criteria have been drawn from a variety of sources (*see* Chapter 4). The standards are broad statements of principle, while the criteria are specific statements that should be assessable.

- **E**, essential practice (if these criteria are not in place then legal and/or professional requirements will not be met, resulting in risk to patients, staff or the public).
- **G**, good practice (standard good practice expected to be in place across the UK).
- **D**, desirable practice (good practice that is not yet standard across the UK).

These standards may not be reproduced or distributed in any form without the written permission of the Royal College of General Practitioners.

Section 1 Service for patients

Accessibility

1   Patients are able to obtain the services of the team at appropriate times and without undue delay.

Criteria	Yes	No	N/A
1.1 **E** Patients with urgent problems are seen on the same day			
1.2 **G** Patients with non-urgent matters are normally seen within 2 working days by any GP or within 7 days by a chosen doctor			
1.3 **G** Patients are not kept waiting unnecessarily in surgery and are informed of the reasons for any delays			
1.4 **G** Patients can contact members of the team directly and arrangements for this are made clear to patients			
1.5 **G** Patients can contact the practice and a team member by telephone during the working day			
1.6 **G** There are sufficient telephone lines and staff to answer them for the size of the practice and the expected demand			
1.7 **E** There is a reliable system to ensure that messages and requests for visits are recorded and that the appropriate doctor or team member receives and acts upon them			
1.8 **E** Patients are visited at home if their condition so requires at the discretion of the GP			
1.9 **G** The reception staff are helpful to patients and facilitate contact with members of the team			

continued

Criteria	Yes	No	N/A

1.10 G The practice is open during its stated opening hours, which are at times likely to be convenient to patients

1.11 E The doctors in the practice are available for their agreed hours and take steps to ensure continuity of care when they are absent and during 'out of hours'

1.12 The practice normally agrees to accept patients requesting to join their list who are eligible to be accepted. It does not discriminate on the grounds of:

E a) race, gender, disability

G b) socialclass, age or medical condition

1.13 G The practice has a policy for removing patients from their list, and if it does so it provides an explanation of the reasons in writing to the patient

Communication

2 The team communicates openly with patients and encourages patients' choice and autonomy.

Criteria	Yes	No	N/A

2.1 G The average length of booked appointments with the doctors and nurses in the practice is not less than 10 minutes

2.2 D In consultations, patients' ideas, concerns and expectations are explored, and information, decisions and responsibility are shared

continued

2.3 E   The practice provides patients with a leaflet that describes the services provided by all members of the team and how patients can obtain them. It also describes patients' rights and responsibilities

2.4 G   Notices and educational displays for patients in the surgery convey clear and informative messages

2.5 G   Information leaflets on a range of topics and health promotion literature are readily available to patients

2.6 E   The team has an agreed procedure for handling patient complaints, and this is advertised to the patients

2.7 E   If the team serves significant groups requiring assistance with communication, interpreter services and translated literature are available

Prescribing

3 The professionals in the team prescribe effectively and economically, and in line with published evidence.

Criteria	Yes	No	N/A
3.1 G The team has developed a formulary for prescribing, and monitors their adherence to it			
3.2 G Patients are given full information about the medications that are prescribed to them			
3.3 G Arrangements for repeat prescribing ensure that all patients receiving regular medications are reviewed at least annually			

Investigations

4 Investigations are used, and the results responded to, appropriately by the team.

Criteria	Yes	No	N/A
4.1 **G** The team has a policy for the appropriate use of investigations, including those for patients with chronic diseases and regular medication. Its use in practice is audited			
4.2 **G** The arrangements for laboratory investigations are reliable, convenient for patients and can include patients confined to their home			
4.3 **E** There is an explicit and reliable system to receive any hospital report or investigation result, to identify the responsible doctor, and to ensure that any necessary action is taken			
4.4 **G** There is an explicit policy for informing patients of the results of their investigations, which is explained to patients			

Preventive health services and health promotion

5   The team identifies the health needs of their population, delivers appropriate preventive health services, and works with their patients, other agencies and their community to promote health.

Criteria	Yes	No	N/A
5.1 E Newly registered patients are offered a consultation to ascertain details of their past medical and family histories, social factors, life style, and measurements of risk factors. These findings are recorded in the medical records			
5.2 G The practice collects information on the factors that put their patients' health at risk, including smoking habit, alcohol intake, physical activity and blood pressure			
5.3 G Patients are given appropriate advice about general health, risk factors including smoking cessation and life style			
5.4 E Patients are offered appropriate vaccinations and immunisations			
5.5 D The team produces a profile of the health needs of their population and identifies strategies for tackling inequalities in health			

Chronic disease care

6 The team manages patients with chronic diseases, including asthma, diabetes, hypertension and arterial disease, in line with modern medical opinion and guidelines.

Criteria	Yes	No	N/A
6.1 **G** The team has developed protocols for the management of chronic diseases, which are used to guide the care that they provide			
6.2 **G** Patients with chronic diseases are offered appropriate education and advice to enable them to control their disease and reduce associated risk factors			
6.3 **G** The team ensures that systematic call and recall of patients on their register is taking place and that they are reviewed regularly, either in hospital or in the practice			
6.4 **G** There is effective communication between the team and hospitals and other professionals caring for their patients			
6.5 **G** The team audits their chronic disease management regularly			

Childrens' health

7   The team provides comprehensive care for children, including immunisations, surveillance and accessible care when they are ill.

Criteria	Yes	No	N/A
7.1 G The roles of the GPs, practice nurses and health visitors in providing care for children in the practice, and the methods of communication between them, are defined and agreed			
7.2 E Children are offered immunisations at the intervals agreed in existing guidelines			
7.3 E Parents are offered full information about immunisations, and their consent and any contraindications to immunisations are recorded clearly and accessibly in the records			
7.4 E Parents hold a record of their children's health, and members of the team offer to complete it			
7.5 E Children's development is assessed at the intervals agreed in existing guidelines and any problems are followed up			
7.6 E Children who are overdue for immunisations or developmental checks are identified and followed up			
7.7 D The team takes steps to enhance parents' ability and confidence to care for their children when they are ill			
7.8 E All clinical team members are aware of the local procedures for child protection and adhere to them			

Mental health services

8   Patients have access to a comprehensive range of mental health services that meets their needs.

Criteria	Yes	No	N/A
8.1 **D** The team has strategies for the detection of patients with depression and alcohol problems			
8.2 **G** Patients with anxiety, depression and problems with alcohol and drugs are able to receive both treatment and non-pharmacological management and support			
8.3 **G** The team participates with the community mental health services in the shared care of patients with chronic mental health problems			
8.4 **E** If a counsellor works in the practice, he or she has appropriate qualifications and continued support			

Family planning and women's health

9   Women patients have access to a comprehensive service that meets accepted professional standards and their needs.

Criteria	Yes	No	N/A
9.1 **G** The rubella immune status of women of childbearing age is established and recorded, and those who require immunisation are offered it			
9.2 **E** Women are called and recalled for cervical cytology in accordance with local policies and there is an agreed policy for identifying and following up non-attenders			

continued

Criteria		Yes	No	N/A
9.3 **G**	Women are offered the choice of a female nurse/doctor to take their smear			
9.4 **G**	The inadequate smear rate is audited regularly and responded to			
9.5 **E**	There is a reliable system for responding to and ensuring follow-up of abnormal smears			
9.6 **G**	Women are clearly informed of the way that they will obtain the result of their smear			
9.7 **G**	The team ensures that women have access to a comprehensive range of family planning services. If some services are not available in the practice women are informed how they can obtain them			
9.8 **G**	The team has an agreed policy for responding appropriately to requests for emergency contraception			
9.9 **G**	The team ensures that family planning services are accessible and acceptable to teenagers			
9.10 **G**	Women who do not attend for breast screening can be identified and encouraged to do so			

Maternity services

10 Women receive maternity services that are based on informed patient choice, accepted professional practice, and that meet their needs.

Criteria	Yes	No	N/A
10.1 **G** The team has an agreed policy for providing preconceptual advice			
10.2 **G** There is an agreed policy for the roles of the GP, community midwife, health visitor and hospital clinics in the provision of ante-natal and post-natal care and for communication between them			
10.3 **G** Women are fully informed and offered a choice about the place of their ante-natal care and delivery			
10.4 **E** Ante-natal care and screening are offered according to current professional guidelines, such as the UKCC Midwives Rules and UKCC Code of Practice			
10.5 **D** Women and their partners have access to parentcraft classes			
10.6 **G** Women are encouraged to breast feed			
10.7 **D** The breast feeding rate is audited			

Continued care at home

11   The team works with social services and other agencies to provide care and support in the community for patients and their carers.

Criteria	Yes	No	N/A
11.1 G Patients requiring care in their home are assessed by members of the team and care is planned and provided to meet their needs			
11.2 G The team works with social services and other agencies to avoid duplication of assessments and to co-ordinate their care			
11.3 G Patients and their carers are offered information and choice about the care they receive			
11.4 G The team works together and with other agencies to provide terminal and palliative care that is comprehensive and meets the needs of patients and their carers			
11.5 D Team members regularly review together the care that they are providing			

Elderly surveillance

12   The needs of elderly patients are assessed by the team and care is planned and provided to meet the needs identified.

Criteria	Yes	No	N/A
12.1 **E** Patients aged 75 or over are offered an annual consultation or home visit to assess their health and needs for care			
12.2 **E** These assessments included sensory functions, mobility, mental condition, physical condition and social environment			
12.3 **G** The conclusions from these assessments are discussed with the patient and their carers if appropriate, and necessary services are requested or provided			
12.4 **D** The needs identified guide the planning and provision of services by the team			

Minor operations

13   The performance of minor operations in the practice conforms to accepted standards of professional practice.

Criteria	Yes	No	N/A
13.1 **E** The premises, equipment and arrangements for sterilisation are appropriate			
13.2 **E** Patients are offered information and choice about any procedures to be performed			
13.3 **D** The practice audits their minor operations against accepted guidelines			

Section 2 The primary care team

Team values

14   The primary care team works together to provide high-quality, continuing, personal and comprehensive care to their patients and their practice population.

Criteria	Yes	No	N/A
14.1 **D** The team is committed to working with individuals, groups and the community to care for people who are ill and to promote health			
14.2 **E** All patients are treated with courtesy and respect for their privacy and dignity			
14.3 **G** Members of the team are committed to working together and respect each others professionalism			
14.4 **D** The team has developed in response to new needs, subjects its work to critical self-scrutiny and continually maintains its skills and widens its horizons			
14.5 **G** Team members accept their obligation to maintain their physical and mental health and keep in bounds their need to be needed			
14.6 **E** All team members maintain patient confidentiality			

Training and continued learning

15   All staff in the team are suitably qualified and maintain their competence for their duties.

Criteria	Yes	No	N/A
15.1 **G** The doctors in the practice have fulfilled the educational requirements to receive the Post Graduate Educational Allowance			
15.2 **G** The practice manager and other staff in the practice have appropriate qualifications and training			
15.3 **E** The team members have appropriate qualifications and training and only carry out treatment for which they are competent			
15.4 **E** Nurses in the team identify their training/educational needs and update their professional practice in accordance with UKCC standards and principles of practice			
15.5 **E** The practice takes reasonable steps to ensure that doctors who are employed as deputies or assistants are qualified and competent to undertake the duties for which they are to be employed			
15.6 **G** The practice gives all members the opportunities and support they require to undertake appropriate training to maintain their competence			

Teamworking

16 The organisation of the team promotes effective communication and teamwork.

Criteria	Yes	No	N/A
16.1 G The doctors, practice staff and other members of the practice team have frequent opportunity to meet informally			
16.2 G Mechanisms for referral and feedback between team members are agreed and effective			
16.3 G There is an agreed mechanism for informing all team members involved when patients are admitted to or discharged from hospital, or when they die			
16.4 G There is an effective means of sharing written communications with team members			
16.5 G Regular team meetings take place to discuss clinical issues and policies			
16.6 G Records are kept of decisions made and actions to be taken at meetings, and these are available to team members			
16.7 G There are written policies covering administrative and clinical procedures that have been discussed and agreed by team members and which are reviewed regularly			
16.8 G There are opportunities for multidisciplinary training for team members			
16.9 G Team members have identified sources of support both within and outside the team			

Records

17   The team keeps adequate records of the illnesses and treatment of patients.

Criteria	Yes	No	N/A
17.1 **E** An entry is made in the record of each patient contact, including visits and telephone advice			
17.2 **E** Entries in the records are complete, accurate and legible			
17.3 **G** The records, hospital letters and investigation reports are filed in date order			
17.4 **G** Referral letters are typewritten, contain all the relevant information, and copies are filed in the patient's record			
17.5 **G** The medication that a patient is receiving is clearly listed in their record			
17.6 **G** Each patient's record contains a summary of significant past and continuing problems, and there is an effective procedure for keeping these updated			
17.7 **G** All clinical members of the team have access to the patient's records and to the practice computer if significant information, e.g. medication, is held there			
17.8 **G** Nursing care plans are held by the patient and are accessible to other team members			

continued

Criteria	Yes	No	N/A
17.9 **E** Patients have access to their records on request in accordance with Data Protection Act and Access to Records Act			
17.10 **G** There are agreed procedures for handling records coming into the practice and for responding promptly to requests to return records to the health authority			
17.11 **E** If the team uses a computer, it is registered under and conforms to the provisions of the Data Protection Act			
17.12 **G** Adequate measures are taken to protect and back up computerised data			
17.13 **G** The practice maintains an age–sex register of its registered population			
17.14 **G** The practice maintains a register of patients with chronic diseases and there are agreed definitions for entering data			

Management

18   The team is managed effectively for the benefit of patients, team members and to meet financial statutory and other responsibilities.

Criteria	Yes	No	N/A
18.1 **G** Responsibilities for management and administration of the team are clearly defined			
18.2 **G** There are regular, minuted meetings of those members of the team with management responsibility			

continued

Criteria	Yes	No	N/A
18.3 **D** The practice operates an explicit management cycle that includes: a profile of the needs of the practice population, a business plan setting objectives and targets for the year, an annual report containing a review of the objectives			
18.4 **D** All members of the team contribute to each stage of the management cycle			
18.5 **D** The team has effective methods of consulting patients about their views of the services provided; for example, patient meetings, patient satisfaction surveys or focus-groups			
18.6 **D** The financial management of the practice includes: defined responsibilities, an annual budget, regular reports of income, expenditure and cash flow, monitoring of claims for items of service, reimbursements and other payments			
18.7 **E** All statutory regulations in relation to staff employment (e.g. equal opportunities, national insurance, PAYE, statutory sick pay) are adhered to and records kept			
18.8 **E** There is an agreed disciplinary procedure that adheres to statutory requirements			
18.9 **G** All staff receive induction and any necessary training, a job description and a contract of employment			

continued

Criteria	Yes	No	N/A
18.10 D All team members are regularly appraised and personal learning plans are agreed			
18.11 G Accurate and complete personnel records are kept			
18.12 G There are rotas for doctors, nurses and practice staff that ensure that an adequate service can be provided for patients at all times			
18.13 E The practice adheres to statutory requirements, including the Health and Safety at Work Act and other regulations covering: training of staff, storage of hazardous substances, storage of drugs, needles, prescriptions, immunisations for team members, employer's liability insurance, disposal of hazardous waste, fire safety, electrical safety			

Quality assurance and audit

19   Regular reviews of performance and audit are an integral part of the work of the team.

Criteria	Yes	No	N/A
19.1 D The team has completed audits that cover a range of topics, including clinical care and practice organisation			
19.2 D The reviews involve all stages of the audit cycle, including agreeing criteria, collecting reliable information, reviewing performance and planning change, and repeating the audit to monitor change			

continued

Criteria	Yes	No	N/A

19.3 D All members of the team contributing to care are involved in conducting audits

19.4 D The team has established mechanisms for the continual monitoring and improvement of the services they provide

Premises

20 The team has sufficient and appropriate accommodation and equipment at the practice premises.

Criteria	Yes	No	N/A

20.1 E The premises are clean, warm, well lit and well maintained

20.2 E The practice premises are accessible to disabled people

20.3 E The practice possesses the equipment and drugs required to deal with serious acute conditions

20.4 E The team members have available all necessary clinical equipment, which is maintained regularly

20.5 G The practice has a library that is accessible to all team members, which contains up-to-date reference books, books relevant to primary care and recent copies of major medical and nursing journals

Index